QUALITY-OF-LIFE RESEARCH ON CHILDREN AND ADOLESCENTS

Edited by

ANNE DANNERBECK

University of Missouri, Columbia, MO, USA

FERRAN CASAS, MARTA SADURNI
and GERMÀ COENDERS

University of Girona, Girona, Spain

Reprinted from *Social Indicators Research*, Volume 66, Nos. 1–2 (April 2004)

KLUWER ACADEMIC PUBLISHERS
DORDRECHT / BOSTON / LONDON

Social Indicators Research Series

Volume 23

This new series aims to provide a public forum for single treatises and collections of papers on social indicators research that are too long to be published in our journal *Social Indicators Research*. Like the journal, the book series deals with statistical assessments of the quality of life from a broad perspective. It welcomes the research on a wide variety of substantive areas, including health, crime, housing, education, family life, leisure activities, transportation, mobility, economics, work, religion and environmental issues. These areas of research will focus on the impact of key issues such as health on the overall quality of life and vice versa. An international review board, consisting of Ruut Veenhoven, Joachim Vogel, Ed Diener, Torbjorn Moum and Wolfgang Glatzer, will ensure the high quality of the series as a whole.

The titles published in this series are listed at the end of this volume.

CONTENTS

A C.I.P. Catalogue record for this book is available from the Library of Congress.

ISBN 1-4020-2311-1

Published by Kluwer Academic Publishers,
P.O. Box 17, 3300 AA Dordrecht, The Netherlands.

Sold and distributed in North, Central and South America
by Kluwer Academic Publishers,
101 Philip Drive, Norwell, MA 02061, U.S.A.

In all other countries, sold and distributed
by Kluwer Academic Publishers,
P.O. Box 322, 3300 AH Dordrecht, The Netherlands.

Printed on acid-free paper

Printed and bound in the Netherlands.

ACKNOWLEDGEMENTS

The impetus for this special volume came from the International Society for Quality of Life Studies 2000 meetings in Girona, Spain. Alex Michalos mentioned to both Ferran Casas (from the University of Girona) and me that such a volume would be well received by the readers. Marta Sadurni (also from the University of Girona) and I, co-chairs of the sessions on child well-being, sat down one day and talked about soliciting manuscripts from conference presenters for a special volume related to the same topic. We noted that separate measurements of life satisfaction among children and adolescents was an emerging area of study. We were pleased that young people were being recognized as assessing their lives differently than adults.

We did not get enough manuscripts from that original solicitation to actually compile a volume. By the time the ISQOLS meetings came around again in Washington, DC in 2001, Ferran Casas had joined us. We announced the manuscript solicitation again and had better response but still not adequate. Then, Scott Huebner (University of South Carolina) stepped in to help identify a number of his colleagues who were working in the area. With his help, we were able to attract a sufficient number of quality papers.

In the review process, Marta, Ferran and I realized that we did not have all the technical expertise needed to critically evaluate some of the analytic methods. Germà Coenders (University of Girona) joined us as a fourth editor.

We are pleased to present to you this compilation of quality of life studies on children and adolescents.

Anne Dannerbeck
University of Missouri

E. SCOTT HUEBNER

RESEARCH ON ASSESSMENT OF LIFE SATISFACTION OF CHILDREN AND ADOLESCENTS

ABSTRACT. Over the years, various psychologists have issued calls for greater attention to a science of positive psychology, which focuses on studying conditions that promote optimal human and societal development. Recent calls (e.g., McCullough and Snyder, 2000; Seligman and Csikszentmihalyi, 2000) have furthered interest in studies of the nature and determinants of the good life. Such a science, along with the creation of prevention and intervention programs informed by the expanded scientific framework, is expected to improve the quality of life for all individuals, not just individuals who are at risk or who already demonstrate psychopathological conditions. To contrast with the previous emphasis on psychopathology, the development of a positive psychology requires constructs and measures that reflect the full range of human functioning, incorporating indicators of high levels of wellness as well as psychopathological functioning. This article discusses one such construct, life satisfaction, that has been studied extensively in adulthood (see Diener et al., 1999), but which has only recently gained attention with children and adolescents (see Bender, 1997; Huebner, 1997). This article reviews life satisfaction assessment research with children and adolescents, specifically with regard to construct validity. In doing so, the following areas are addressed: models of life satisfaction; convergent validity; discriminant validity; relationships with other well-being measures; relationships with external, environmental circumstances; relationships with demographic variables; cultural factors; group differences on life satisfaction measures; predictive relationships; and stability of life satisfaction reports. Conclusions regarding the validity of the life satisfaction construct are formulated. Recommendations for future research are also discussed.

KEY WORDS: adolescents, assessment, children, life satisfaction, quality of life

According to some authors, psychologists have disproportionately focused on the study of psychological ill-being (McCullough and Snyder, 2000; Seligman and Csikszentmihalyi, 2000). These authors suggest that psychologists should pay greater attention to the complementary study of psychological well-being, including the development and enhancement of human strengths and environmental resources. Although comprehensive taxonomies of human

Social Indicators Research **66:** 3–33, 2004.

strengths are in their early stages of development (see Seligman, 2002), most taxonomies include individuals' perceptions of the quality of their lives (i.e., life satisfaction).

Research regarding child and adolescent judgments of their life satisfaction has received increasing attention in a variety of areas, including regular and special education (e.g., Crocker, 2000; Huebner, 1997). As early as 1986, Landesman (1986) noted that quality of life and personal life satisfaction were the new buzz words in the field of mental disabilities. Current researchers in public health (e.g., Day and Jankey, 1996; Valois et al., 2001) have extended quality of life concepts to health promotion efforts for *all* individuals. Although early work was primarily aimed at adults, work has begun to extend to children and adolescents as well.

Quality of life has been studied from two major perspectives: objective and subjective. Objective measures focus on external, quantifiable conditions such as income levels, access to medical resources, and recreational opportunities. In contrast, subjective measures focus on internal evaluations of life circumstances (e.g., satisfaction judgments, emotions). The relationships between the two sets of measures have been quite modest, leading most researchers to infer that each approach contains unique, complementary information that is relevant to understanding quality of life. The strengths and weaknesses of each approach are considered thoroughly by Diener and Suh (1997).

Quality of life holds a central position in the evaluation of psychosocial, educational, and medical services for individuals with and without disabilities (Cowen, 1991; Felce and Perry, 1996). With individuals with disabilities, quality of life is a crucial outcome variable because of the important role of support services in affecting persons' lives. As services for children and youth have become more multifaceted, with an increased range of intended outcomes, the requirements for evaluation have extended to quality of life concerns. For example, numerous authors have argued that public school reform efforts should extend beyond academic outcomes to incorporate affective outcomes as well (e.g., Hegarty, 1994; Huebner and McCullough, 2000; Phillips, 1993). The relevant indicators of subjective quality of life in the school context have not been agreed upon, however, life satisfaction judgments have been shown to be relevant to school functioning (Huebner and Alderman, 1993; Huebner et al., 2000).

Life satisfaction measures are also consistent with an expanded interest in defining and measuring health, including mental health, as more than simply the absence of psychopathological symptoms. For example, Kazdin (1993) argued that the mental health of youth encompassed two domains: the absence of dysfunction and optimal functioning in psychological domains. Similarly, Seligman and Csikszentmihalyi (2000) have issued a call for a science of positive psychology to complement psychology's historical emphasis on psychopathological conditions. Theory and measurement related to optimal well-being require adaptive constructs and measures that tap the presence of personal strengths, not just the absence of psychopathological symptoms. The life satisfaction construct fulfills this requirement as it incorporates the full range of satisfaction (e.g., from very low to neutral to very high). In this manner, life satisfaction reports can be sensitive to subtle changes above the neutral point as well as below the neutral point (Kamman et al., 1984). The relationship between life dissatisfaction and a diagnosis of psychopathology is not necessarily concordant, however. For example, a person may be dissatisfied with her/his life without showing psychopathological symptoms, which may be adaptive given the experience of highly undesirable environmental circumstances (Greenspoon and Saklofske, 2000).

Global life satisfaction has been defined as a cognitive evaluation of one's life as a whole (Shin and Johnson, 1984). Although affect can influence life satisfaction reports, life satisfaction is distinguished from transitory affective states. Emotions refer to specific on-line reactions to specific events that occur in people's lives, such as anger, joy, anxiety, and so forth. Life satisfaction reports typically refer to more general, enduring background appraisals encompassing one's overall life or major facets of one's life (Diener et al., 1999; Lazarus, 1991). Although experiences of frequent positive emotions, infrequent negative emotions, and life satisfaction tend to intercorrelate, suggesting a higher-order subjective well-being factor, affective and life satisfaction reports can diverge over time and demonstrate different determinants (see Diener, 1994).

Although the importance of specific facets of life satisfaction has been debated (Andrews and Robinson, 1991; Chamberlain, 1988; Seligson et al., 2003), life satisfaction has been studied from a multidimensional perspective as well. For example, measures of a variety of domains have been developed, such as satisfaction with school life, friends, self, and so forth. Research using both strategies has been fruitful; however, this review focuses mostly on global life satisfaction research.

Life satisfaction has been studied from the perspective that it is an important outcome in and of itself (Diener et al., 1999). Considerable research has been devoted to attempting to understand the determinants of a person's perceptions of the good life. However, studies have also suggested that life satisfaction judgments operate not just as a byproduct of particular life experiences and personal characteristics, but that life satisfaction judgments also in turn influence crucial processes and behaviors. For example, the importance of maintaining positive levels of subjective well-being has been articulated by Frederickson (1998). She provides evidence that positive subjective experiences serve to broaden and build resources, regulate negative affective experiences, and protect health. Studies of correlates of life satisfaction in adults suggest that positive life satisfaction is linked with positive social interactions, broadened perception and creativity, active involvement in community and political organizations, fewer physical complaints, and longer lives (Veenhoven, 1988). On the other side of the coin, low levels of life satisfaction have been linked with negative adaptive outcomes, such as depression (Lewinsohn et al., 1991), interpersonal rejection (Furr and Funder, 1998), aggressive behavior (Suldo and Huebner, 2003; Valois et al., 2001), and alcohol (Newcomb et al., 1986; Raphael et al., 1996) and chemical abuse (Zullig et al., 2001).

Although research with children and adolescents is just beginning, the preliminary findings have been encouraging. The purpose of this article is to provide a review of the extant research on assessment of the life satisfaction of children and adolescents. This research provides valuable information that informs the conceptualization, measurement, and importance of life satisfaction. Specifically, the review addresses the following issues: (1) theoretical models of life satisfaction; (2) convergent validity; (3) discriminant validity; (4) relationships with other well-being measures (5) relationships with external, environmental circumstances; (6) relationships with demographic variables; (7) cultural factors; (8) group differences on life satisfaction scales; (9) predictive relationships; and (10) stability of life satisfaction reports. Taken together, the findings have important implications for future investigation of the life satisfaction construct, particularly vis-a-vis the positive psychology movement

LITERATURE REVIEW

Theoretical Models of Life Satisfaction

Life satisfaction measures have been derived from a number of alternative models of life satisfaction. The models can be organized within three major conceptual frameworks, including unidimensional (i.e., global or general life satisfaction) and multidimensional ones. The two unidimensional models converge in the assumption that a single, total score can represent different levels of life satisfaction. The models diverge with respect to the method of aggregation. The general model assumes that the total score should consist of the sum (weighted or unweighted) of satisfaction reports across different life domains, such as satisfaction with friends, family, school, neighborhood, and so forth. Measures based on this method require that the authors have included the crucial domains that contribute to overall life satisfaction. In contrast, the global model assumes that life satisfaction judgments are best assessed through items that are context-free (e.g., I have a good life vs. I have a good *family* life). In this manner, respondents are free to derive their responses based on their own, unique criteria rather than having the criteria imposed by the researcher (Pavot and Diener, 1993).

The multidimensional framework deemphasizes the assessment of global or general life satisfaction, focusing more on the derivation of profiles of life satisfaction judgments across key life domains. As one example, Huebner et al. (1998) proposed a hierarchical life satisfaction model in which five specific second-order domains (school, family, friends, self, living environment) are included under a general life satisfaction factor. Some authors have proposed multidimensional models in which domain-specific satisfaction reports are moderated by an importance rating given to each domain, although research has not provided support for the incremental validity of importance ratings with children (Seligson et al., 2003).

A number of measures of life satisfaction have been developed for use with children and adolescents. Such measures are necessary to take into account differences between adults and children, including differences related to intellectual development, psychosocial maturity, interests, reading ability, and life circumstances (e.g., autonomy). These measures include the Brief Multidimensional Students' Life Satisfaction Scale (BMSLSS: Seligson et al., 2003), Comprehensive Quality of Life Scale-Adolescent Version (COM-QOL: Cummins, 1997; see also Gullone and Cummins, 1999), Multidimensional Students' Life Satisfaction Scale (MSLSS: Huebner, 1994a), Perceived Life Satisfaction Scale (PLSS: Adelman et al., 1989), Students' Life Satisfaction Scale (SLSS: Huebner, 1991a), Quality of Life Profile-Adolescent Version (QOLP-Q: Raphael et al., 1996). Reviews of the psychometric properties of some of these measures can be found in Bender (1997) and Gilman and Huebner (2001).

Relationships among Life Satisfaction Measures

Several investigations have explored the relationship between pairs of different measures of life satisfaction. In a sample of high school students, Dew and Huebner (1994) obtained a correlation of 0.58 between the SLSS, which purports to measure global life satisfaction, and the PLSS, which purports to measure general life satisfaction. The SLSS also demonstrated a correlation of 0.62 with a widely used one-item life satisfaction index (Andrews and Withey, 1976) in a sample of elementary school students (Huebner, 1991a) and demonstrated a correlation of 0.66 with the BMSLSS in sample of middle school students (Seligson et al., 2003). Huebner (1994) also reported that the SLSS correlated 0.57 with the Happiness and Life Satisfaction subscale of the Piers-Harris Self-Concept Scale (Piers, 1984), although noting that the subscale is not a pure measure of life satisfaction given that happiness and life satisfaction are theoretically and empirically distinct (Lucas et al., 1996). In a study of Canadian children in grades 3–8, Greenspoon and Saklofske (1997) found a correlation of 0.61 between the total score of the

MSLSS and a one-item index of overall life satisfaction constructed specifically for their study. Finally, using latent trait methodology, Laughlin and Huebner (2002) obtained an r-square of 0.88 between global life satisfaction, as measured by the SLSS, and general life satisfaction, as measured by the MSLSS domains, in a sample of adolescent students in grades 6–8.

Convergent validity has also been studied through studies of the correspondence between self-reports of life satisfaction and those of knowledgeable others (e.g., parents, friends). For comparison purposes, Lucas et al. (1996) reported a mean correlation of 0.41 between college students' self and other-ratings using the Satisfaction with Life Scale (Diener et al., 1985). Using the SLSS, Dew and Huebner (1994) obtained a correlation of 0.48 between the global ratings of high school students and their parents, and Gilman and Huebner (1997) obtained a correlation of 0.54 between middle school students and their parents. Based upon a study of the MSLSS with adolescents, Huebner et al. (2002) reported correlations between parent and adolescent reports, ranging from 0.41 to 0.55, across five domains of life satisfaction. These self-other correlations compare favorably to the meta-analytic findings of Achenbach et al. (1987), in which the mean correlation between the (behavioral) ratings of self and other informants was 0.22.

Although the development of life satisfaction measures appropriate for children and youth is just beginning, these studies provide evidence of convergent validity across various measures. Nevertheless, the moderate magnitude of some of the correlations suggests the need for further inquiry. These correlations likely reflect some attenuation due to the different theoretical models underlying the various instruments.

Discriminant Validity

Although convergence between different measures of life satisfaction is important, discriminant validity is particularly crucial because much of the life satisfaction/quality of life literature has developed from research traditions other than psychology (e.g., sociology, gerontology). Discriminant validity reflects the extent to which a construct is differentiable from other subjective quality of life constructs that it subsumes or to which it is related. For example, in Huebner's (1997) model, general life satisfaction has been distinguished from one of its theorized subcomponents, that is, self-esteem or self-satisfaction. Empirical support for the separability of the life satisfaction and self-esteem measures has been provided by exploratory and confirmatory factor analytic studies (Huebner, 1994b; Huebner et al., 1999; Terry and Huebner, 1995). In addition to demonstrating that children are able to reliably differentiate the two constructs, Huebner et al. (1999) demonstrated a pattern of differential correlates for the two constructs. As one example, adolescents' self-perceived physical attractiveness is a strong correlate of self-esteem, but only a modest correlate of life satisfaction.

Life satisfaction has also been differentiated from frequency of positive and negative affect in children (Huebner, 1991c) and adolescents (Huebner and Dew, 1996). Patterns of differential correlations among the three constructs and demographic variables (gender, ethnicity, and socioeconomic status) were shown with adolescents (Huebner and Dew, 1996).

Similarly, life satisfaction has been shown to measure something different from indices of psychopathology. A conjoint factor analysis of the SLSS and Youth Self Report (short form) of the Child Behavior Checklist (Achenbach and Edelbrock, 1991) with adolescents revealed three clearly distinct factors of internalizing disorders, externalizing disorders, and global life satisfaction (Suldo, 2001). Shek (1998) demonstrated divergence across time between the development of psychopathological disorders and life satisfaction in adolescents. Furthermore, life satisfaction has been differentiated from depression, although most of the work has been done with adults. For example, Lewinsohn et al. (1991) demonstrated a prodromal relationship with depression in which declining life satisfaction reports predicted the onset of clinical depression in a longitudinal study. However, studies of children and adolescents consistently report no gender differences in life satisfaction for children and youth across grades 3–12 (Ash and Huebner, 2001; Dew and Huebner, 1994; Huebner, 1991a, b; Terry and Huebner, 1995) in contrast to robust gender differences in depression in children and adolescents (Compas et al., 1997; Hammen and Rudolph, 1996). Finally, Greenspoon and Saklofske (2001) demonstrated that children (grades 3–6) reporting low life satisfaction (along with high psychopathology) could be distinguished meaningfully from children reporting low life satisfaction (along with low psychopathology) on a number of dimensions, supporting the distinctiveness of the life satisfaction construct.

Life satisfaction reports have demonstrated non-significant relationships with a number of more distinct psychological constructs. Life satisfaction reports of children have been differentiated from social desirability responding (Huebner, 1991a). Also, life satisfaction has been shown to be separate from measures of intellectual ability (Huebner and Alderman, 1993), school grades (Huebner, 1991b), and academic self-efficacy (Gilman and Huebner, 1997).

Relationships with Other Well-Being Measures

Life satisfaction reports of children and adolescents are related to a wide array of psychosocial variables in meaningful ways. Summaries of studies of psychosocial correlates are presented in Table I. This nomological network includes significant negative relationships with a variety of indicators of maladaptive functioning and significant positive relationships with indicators of adaptive functioning. These studies show that individual differences in life satisfaction are related to affective, cognitive, and behavioral functioning of children and youth. Correlates include temperament, coping styles, cognitive attributions, as well as intrapersonal (e.g., drug use, depression) and interpersonal (e.g., aggressive behavior, loneliness) factors. Specifically, high life satisfaction in children and youth is related to extraverted temperament, active coping, internal locus of control, positive self-concept and purpose in life, participation in meaningful, prosocial activities, and lower likelihood of involvement with drugs and/or alcohol and psychopathological (externalizing and internalizing) behavior.

Environmental Experiences

As would be expected, life satisfaction judgments of children and adolescents have been linked with environmental experiences. McCullough et al. (2000) found that ongoing daily positive and negative experiences (e.g., chronic family discord) correlated 0.39 and –0.34 respectively with global life satisfaction in a sample of

TABLE I

Studies of correlates of life satisfaction of children and/or adolescents

Study	Participants	Measure	Correlates
Adelman et al., 1989	47 children referred by school to mental health center, ages 7 to 16 515 students ages 9 to 19 (included above sample)	Perceived Life Satisfaction Scale	Negatively correlated with depression Positively correlated with perceived control at school
Ash and Huebner, 2002	152 high school students	Students' Life Satisfaction Scale	Positively correlated with positive life events, environmental resources, and internal locus of control
Dew and Huebner, 1994	222 high school students	Students' Life Satisfaction Scale	Positively correlated with internal locus of control, global self-esteem and self-concept areas: physical abilities, physical appearance, opposite-sex peer relations, same-sex peer relations, honesty-trustworthiness, parent relations, emotional stability
Fogle et al., in press	160 middle school students	Students' Life Satisfaction Scale	Positively correlated with extraversion and social self-efficacy Negatively correlated with neuroticism
Gilman, 2001	321 students, grades 9–12	Multidimensional Students' Life Satisfaction Scale	Positive correlated with social interest and participation in extra curricular activities

TABLE I

Continued

Study	Participants	Measure	Correlates
Greenspoon and Saklofske, 1997	314 children, grades 3–8	Multidimensional Students' Life Satisfaction Scale	Positively correlated with social skills and leadership Negatively correlated with: withdrawal, anxiety, depression, school problems
Grob et al., 1999	Cross-cultural sample of adolescents	Berne Questionnaire on Adolescents' Well-Being	Negatively correlated with strain and emotion-oriented coping Positively correlated with global control expectancy and problem-oriented coping
Gullone and Cummins, 1999	264 adolescents, 12–18 years old	Comprehensive Quality of Life Scale-Subjective	Negatively correlated with anxiety
Huebner, 1991	79 middle school students	Students' Life Satisfaction Scale	Negatively correlated with anxiety, locus of control and neuroticism Positively correlated with extraversion and self-esteem
Huebner and Alderman, 1993	28 children at risk program for academic failure, learning or emotional problems, 3rd–6th grade	Students' Life Satisfaction Scale	Negatively correlated with depression, loneliness and social dissatisfaction Positively correlated with self- esteem

TABLE I

Continued

Study	Participants	Measure	Correlates
	28 3rd–5th graders		Negatively correlated with depression, loneliness and social dissatisfaction Positively correlated with self- esteem
	43 students grades 2–6, 10 students 7–9, referred or undergoing re-evaluation		Negatively correlated with teacher-rated behavior problems
Huebner et al., 2000	321 high school students	Students' Life Satisfaction Scale	Negatively correlated with locus of control, depression, anxiety, social stress, sense of inadequacy (n.s. at Time 2), atypicality, sensation seeking (n.s. at Time 2), attitude to school (n.s. at Time 2), attitude to teacher (n.s. at Time 2) Positively correlated with self-esteem, relations with parents and interpersonal relations
Leung and Leung, 1992	1156 Chinese students, 7th to 9th grade	5-item life satisfaction scale	Positively correlated with academic ability, physical ability, social ability, physical appearance, general self-concept, relationship with parents, relationship with school

TABLE I

Continued

Study	Participants	Measure	Correlates
Magen, 1996	1094 adolescents, ages 14–15, Israeli Jews, Israeli Moslem-Arabs, Christian Americans	Positive Experience Questionnaire	Positively correlated with peer and parent orientation
Man, 1991	1906 Hong Kong students, ages 13–16	26 domain life satisfaction scale	Positively correlated with parent orientation and participation in prosocial activity
Maton, 1990	60 urban black males (ages 15–19) and 32 pregnant adolescents (mean age = 17.0)	Satisfaction with Life Scale	Positively correlated with school status, meaningful instrumental activity, support-parents and support-friends
McCullough et al., 2000	92 high school students	Students' Life Satisfaction Scale	Positively correlated with positive major life events and daily events Negatively correlated with negative major life events and daily events
McKnight et al., 2002	1201 middle and high school students	Students' Life Satisfaction Scale	Positively correlated with extraversion Negatively correlated with stressful life events, externalizing, and internalizing behavior

TABLE I

Continued

Study	Participants	Measure	Correlates
Petito and Cummins, 2000	279 adolescents, ages 12 to 17	Comprehensive Quality of Life Scale-Subjective	Positively correlated with primary control, secondary control, perceived social support and authoritative parenting
Sam, 1998	506 adolescents with immigrant back-grounds living in Norway	Satisfaction with Life-Scale	Positively correlated with sense of mastery
Seligson et al., 2003	221 middle school students	Brief Multidimensional Students' Life Satisfaction	Positively correlated with positive affect Negatively correlated with negative affect
Shek, 1992	2,150 Chinese students, ages 11–20	Purpose in Life Scale B Quality of Existence	Positively correlated with self-perception and ego strength Negatively correlated with general health problems, state anxiety, trait anxiety, depression, chronic, and acute somatic complaints
Shek, 1997	429 Chinese adolescents, ages 12–16	Satisfaction With Life Scale	Positively correlated with paternal ratings, maternal ratings and child ratings of family functioning
Shek, 1998	378 Chinese adolescents, ages 12–16	Satisfaction with Life Scale	Negatively correlated with psychological symptoms

TABLE I

Continued

Study	Participants	Measure	Correlates
Smith et al., 1987	80 students, 9–18 years of age	Perceived Life Satisfaction Scale	Positively correlated with parent behavior ratings, school attitudes, anger control, control satisfaction, goals satisfaction, happiness
Terry and Huebner, 1994	183 students, grades 3–5	Students' Life Satisfaction Scale	Positively correlated with self-concept domains: reading, physical appearance, physical abilities, math, general-school, peers, general-self and parent
Valois et al., 2001	5032 high school students	Brief Multidimensional Students' Life Satisfaction Scale	Related negatively to alcohol and chemical use
Verkuyten, 1986	261 adolescents, 13–16 years of age from the Netherlands	Cantril measure	Positively correlated with positive hedonic affect
Young et al., 1995	640 students, ages 12–16	Five-item Likert scale	Positively correlated with perception of parental closeness and intrinsic support
Zullig et al., 2001	5032 high school students	Brief Multidimensional Students' Life Satisfaction Scale	Related negatively to aggressive behavior (e.g., carrying a weapon, physical fighting)

high school students. Additionally, they found modest to moderate correlations between life satisfaction and acute major positive (r = 0.30) and negative (r = –0.22) life events (e.g., death of a relative). In a different sample of adolescents, Ash and Huebner (2001) found similar correlations between life experiences and life satisfaction. Chronic stressors, such as school (r = –0.41), friends (r = –0.36), and family (r = –0.33), demonstrated the most significant correlations. Also, children's life satisfaction is associated with living in commercial areas in inner cities (Homel and Burns, 1989).

Looking more specifically at particular family behaviors on adolescents' life satisfaction, Young et al. (1995) found that intrinsic (versus extrinsic) support behaviors of parents were related to adolescents' satisfaction. Additionally, Petito and Cummins (2000) and Suldo (2001) also showed significant, positive associations between authoritative parenting behavior, social support, and adolescents' life satisfaction reports.

Research by Ash and Huebner (2001) also supported a cognitive mediational model of life satisfaction, in which the relationship between negative life experiences and life satisfaction was mediated by a generalized external locus of control. Adverse environmental experiences appeared to disrupt adolescents' perceptions of control, which in turn related to reduced life satisfaction. Taken together, the findings suggest that although an individual's life experiences are meaningfully associated with life satisfaction judgments, life experiences do not provide a complete explanation of the association.

Demographic Relationships

Judgments of satisfaction with life as a whole do not appear to be strongly related to demographic variables. Studies have *not* demonstrated robust differences in global life satisfaction related to age or grade level (Dew and Huebner, 1994; Huebner, 1991a; Huebner et al., 2000), although some studies have demonstrated some differences in levels of frequency of positive affect. For example, Greene (1990) found higher positive affect among elementary age children compared to middle and senior high school students.

Global life satisfaction is unrelated to gender in children (grade 3 and above) and adolescents (Dew and Huebner, 1994; Huebner, 1991a, b; Huebner and Alderman, 1993; Huebner et al., 2000). Boys and girls appear equally satisfied with their lives as a whole, despite differences in related experiences, such as depression (Hammen and Rudolph, 1996).

The relationships between race and global life satisfaction have been mixed. In large studies of elementary (Huebner, 1996) and secondary students (Huebner et al., 2000), no differences in overall life satisfaction were demonstrated between African-Americans and Caucasians. However, African-American students reported overall lower life satisfaction in smaller studies of elementary (Terry and Huebner, 1994) and secondary level students (Dew and Huebner, 1994). The relationship between race and life satisfaction may be confounded with socioeconomic status effects (SES). Findings related to SES have also been found to be mixed (Ash and Huebner, 2001), although effects may be stronger for individuals in environments characterized by extreme poverty (Cummins, 2001; Diener and Diener, 1996).

Overall, the findings have suggested modest relationships at best between global life satisfaction and demographic variables. These findings are consistent with those obtained with adults (Diener and Myers, 1995; Diener et al., 1999) and have led to the conclusion that the effects of demographic variables are likely mediated by psychological processes, such as coping styles and differences in goal orientations (Diener et al., 1999).

Group Differences

Expected group differences have been found on measures of overall life satisfaction. Compared to normal children and/or youth, lower global or general satisfaction has been reported for special education students (Smith et al., 1987), students referred for mental health services (Adelman et al., 1989), students with serious emotional disturbance (Huebner and Alderman, 1993), and violent and non-violent adjudicated youth (Crenshaw, 1998). The findings regarding overall life satisfaction provide additional support for the life satisfaction construct.

Assessments using multidimensional measures have also revealed useful findings. In a study of adolescents with mild mental disabilities, the global life satisfaction ratings of adolescent students with mild mental disabilities did not differ from those of normal adolescents. However, differences were found on particular domains of life satisfaction (Brantley et al., 2002). Specifically, adolescents with mild mental disabilities indicated high satisfaction with school experiences and lower satisfaction with friendships compared to comparison peers. Similarly, Griffin and Huebner (2000) observed differences in satisfaction with peer friendships on the MSLSS between adolescents with serious emotional disturbance and normal adolescents. The differences in the specific domains of satisfaction suggest potential practical implications with respect to the development and evaluation of contextualized health promotion programs for children and youth (e.g., see Frisch et al., 1992; Huebner et al., 1998).

Cultural Factors

Studies of adults have demonstrated the influence of cultural and societal factors on life satisfaction (Diener, 2000). However, few studies of cultural factors and life satisfaction have been conducted with children or youth to date. As a prerequisite to studying possible differences in the nomological networks of life satisfaction across cultures and nations, a few studies have addressed measurement equivalence across particular groups. For example, Huebner and Dew (1993) addressed the possibility of test bias in the SLSS. They found equivalence of the factor structure and criterion-related validity across African-American and Caucasian adolescent students in the USA. Similarly, Huebner (1995) obtained comparable results with the SLSS across African-American and Caucasian elementary school students.

Studies of multidimensional life satisfaction reports have also been supportive of cross-cultural comparability. Casas et al. (2001) demonstrated the factorial validity of a Catalan version of the 5-domain MSLSS with a sample of adolescent students in Spain. Also, in a study spanning three age groups (elementary, middle and senior high) of students, Park (2000) found factorial comparability of life satisfaction reports on the MSLSS across Korean and American students.

Although considerable additional research is needed, these studies provide promising support for the further study of life satisfaction across cultures and nations.

Predictive Relationships

Only a few studies have investigated the predictive utility of life satisfaction ratings of children or adolescents. In one study, Shek (1998) found that lower levels of life satisfaction predicted an increase in the general psychological symptoms of adolescents one year later. In another study, Huebner, Funk and Gilman (2000) demonstrated relationships between global life satisfaction ratings of adolescents and several clinical and adaptive scales on the Behavior Assessment System for Children taken one year later (BASC: Reynolds and Kamphaus, 1992). Global life satisfaction reports predicted a number of BASC Clinical subscales (e.g., Depression (r = –0.39), Anxiety (r = –0.33), Social Stress (r = –0.50)) as well as the BASC Adaptive subscales (e.g., Relations with Parents (r = 0.38), Self-Esteem (r = 0.22)). The similarity in the cross-sectional and longitudinal correlation patterns offered credence to the notion that global life satisfaction reports of adolescents represent more than a transitory state of happiness. Finally, Suldo and Huebner (in press) demonstrated that global life satisfaction reports of adolescents not only predicted increased externalizing behavior one year later, but also moderated the development of subsequent externalizing problems in relation to increasing stressful life events. That is, adolescents with positive life satisfaction levels (vs. adolescents who were dissatisfied with their lives) were less likely to develop later externalizing problems in the face of adverse life events. This latter study provided the strongest evidence that life satisfaction operates as a protective psychological strength against the effects of stressful life events in adolescents. Nevertheless, understanding of the meaning and implications of the life satisfaction construct and measures would be greatly enhanced by additional longitudinal investigations.

Stability of Life Satisfaction Reports

Researchers have theorized that life satisfaction reports comprise both state and trait components (e.g., Diener, 1994). Considerable research with adults has been consistent with such theory. Preliminary research investigating the stability of global life satisfaction reports of children and adolescents has also been supportive. Research with the SLSS has demonstrated a two-week test-retest reliability of 0.74 in a sample of 4th through 8th grade students (Huebner, 1991a), a four-week coefficient of 0.64 in a sample of middle schoolers (Gilman and Huebner, 1997), and a one-year coefficient of 0.53 in a sample of high schoolers (Huebner, Funk and Gilman, 2000). With a sample of Canadian students in grades 3–8, Greenspoon and Saklofske reported a one-month stability coefficient of 0.78 for the total (general) score on the MSLSS. Using the PLSS, test-retest coefficients of 0.63 and 0.73 were reported for an unspecified time frame in sample of special and regular education students respectively (Adelman, Taylor and Nelson, 1989).

Studies of multidimensional life satisfaction reports on an adolescent version of the MSLSS have yielded two-week coefficients ranging from 0.85 to 0.93, with a 0.94 for the total score (Dew, Huebner and Laughlin, 2001). Also, four-week coefficients on the MSLSS have ranged from 0.53 to 0.81 (total score = 0.91) in a study with middle school students (Huebner et al., 1998) and 0.59 to 0.78 (total score = 0.78) in a study with elementary and middle school students (Greenspoon and Saklofske, 1997).

The sensitivity of life satisfaction measures to psychosocial intervention has also been demonstrated. Gilman and Handwerk (2001) demonstrated changes in the life satisfaction of a middle school sample related to placement in a residential treatment program. Also, Farrell et al. (in press) demonstrated changes in middle schoolers' life satisfaction following a conflict resolution program. Taken together, studies of global and domain-based satisfaction suggest that child and adolescent life satisfaction reports demonstrate moderate levels of stability, reflecting a somewhat enduring trait-like component, but also sensitivity to changing life circumstances.

CONCLUSIONS

Based on this review, the following conclusions appear warranted regarding children and youth (ages 8–18).

1. Alternative models of life satisfaction of children and youth have been proposed, but have not been rigorously tested against one another.

2. Although the development of life satisfaction scales appropriate for children and adolescents has only recently been undertaken, there is support for the convergent validity of life satisfaction measures.
3. There is developing support for discriminant validity. Life satisfaction appears to be related to, but separable from, a variety of psychological well-being constructs, such as self-esteem, positive affect, and negative affect. Measures of life satisfaction are also distinguishable from measures of psychopathological conditions.
4. Life satisfaction measures show a meaningful nomological network of relations with a variety of important psychosocial variables.
5. Environmental events and experiences relate moderately to life satisfaction reports.
6. Demographic relationships appear to be of limited practical significance in life's satisfaction reports, except perhaps in the case of populations suffering from extreme poverty.
7. Life satisfaction measures differentiate several groups of children (e.g., students with emotional disabilities, adjudicated youth). However, multidimensional measures may offer a more complete assessment for potential applied purposes than unidimensional measures for some groups.
8. Life satisfaction measures have shown promising evidence of equivalence across race and cultures to date.
9. Additional work needs to be done with respect to the predictive utility of life satisfaction reports, however, preliminary research is promising.
10. Life satisfaction measures exhibit moderate stability; they reflect more than the influence of transitory affective states.

Additional research is needed to specify the precise meaning and boundaries of the life satisfaction construct. Nevertheless, life satisfaction appears to be a useful psychological construct that is related to, but separable from, a variety of well-being constructs. Global life satisfaction does not represent an isolated characteristic or appraisal tendency of children and/or youth, but has broad implications for their intrapersonal and interpersonal adaptation in a variety of life contexts. Although related to traditional mental health constructs, life satisfaction encompasses the full range of subjective appraisals from very negative to very positive. Psychometrically sound measures of life satisfaction should thus complement well-being measures that are limited to negative well-being indicators, such as reports of psychopathological symptoms. Given such differentiation, life satisfaction studies should contribute to the development of a science of positive psychology as it is extended to children and adolescents. The study of positive life satisfaction should have considerable heuristic value in attempts to explain and promote positive health outcomes. Additionally, pending appropriate research, life satisfaction measures have many potential applied uses, including program development and evaluation applications at the individual and systems levels (Frisch et al., 1992; Frisch, 1998; Huebner et al. 1998).

In summary, the study of life satisfaction of *adults* has grown into a major area of research in the social sciences (Diener, 1994). The studies reviewed herein support the notion that life satisfaction is a meaningful and important variable for children and adolescents (from about age 8) as well. Although much additional research is needed, life satisfaction measures appear to demonstrate substantial construct validity to date. Thus, these studies provide considerable empirical support for encouraging the further study of life satisfaction among children and adolescents.

IMPLICATIONS FOR RESEARCH

Future life satisfaction research needs to address several important concerns. First, the emergence of theory-directed research would advance the field. Although there is much to be said for exploratory studies in this early stage of development of life satisfaction research with children and adolescents, the articulation of theories informed particularly by knowledge of child and adolescent development is crucial for further development. Recommendations for closer connections between theory and research in life satisfaction work with adults have been made (e.g., Diener, 1984, 1994). The need for such recommendations is even more apparent in research with children and adolescents. To this date, few theory-based studies have appeared in the child and adolescent literature. Theoretical refinement of the construct of life satisfaction is a prerequisite to advances in scale development.

Second, life satisfaction measures for children and youth are also in the early stages of development. Although preliminary work with self-report measures is promising, it is limited in several ways. For example, it is limited in that measures need to be more rigorously evaluated. As noted by Gilman and Huebner (2000), extant measures would benefit from more attention to basic psychometric properties, such as normative samples, reliability, and validity. Research is also sorely needed with respect to the influence of response distortions, importance ratings, developmental changes, cultural differences, and disabilities. For another example, although self-report measures have demonstrated some validity, research incorporating non-self-report measures would enhance the generalizability of findings. As noted by Diener et al. (1999), when non-self-report measures converge with self-report measures, greater confidence will be provided for the conclusions. When non-self-report measures diverge from self-report measures, researchers will develop greater knowledge of the complexity of life satisfaction. Diener (1994) provides a comprehensive discussion of possible alternative measures of life satisfaction, such as measures based on biological indices, facial expressions, experience sampling, and cognitions (e.g., memory for positive experiences).

Studies of child and adolescent life satisfaction have been limited largely to one-shot correlational studies. Although studies of the correlates of life satisfaction have merit, an important next step in the advancement of research would involve studies of the predictive validity of life satisfaction scales. Studies, such as those by Suldo and Huebner (in press) and Lewinsohn et al. (1991), in which low life satisfaction was shown to precede the occurrence of psychopathology, provide much needed information regarding the directionality of life satisfaction effects as well as the potential usefulness of life satisfaction scales in clinical situations. Thus, longitudinal research offers considerable promise for clarifying the nature and implications of child and adolescent life satisfaction reports.

Similarly, studies of the usefulness of life satisfaction reports as sensitive treatment indicators would also enhance the knowledge base in this area. Although some studies suggest that life satisfaction reports may serve as useful outcome measures (e.g. Farrell et al., in press; Gilman and Handwerk, 2001), much additional work needs to be done in this area. In addition to articulating numerous potential uses with adults in applied situations, Frisch et al.'s (2001) research suggests excellent strategies for treatment sensitivity research that would be applicable to children.

Finally, cross-cultural research is also needed. Although few cross-national and/or cross-cultural studies of children and adolescents have been conducted, research with adults has shown robust differences in the nature of satisfaction across different cultural groups. For example, the strong relationship between self-esteem and life satisfaction found in individualistic countries is considerably weaker in collectivistic countries. Cultures also differ with regard to their views of the world as positive and controllable as well as in their norms for expressing negative emotions and cognition (Diener et al., 1998; Grob et al., 1999). For example, Lee and Seligman (1997) reported that white American college students more often attributed success to themselves and failure to other people and circumstances whereas Chinese students demonstrated the opposite pattern. Thus, more research is needed to assess the possibility of differential construct validity of life satisfaction of children and youth across different groups within and across nations.

REFERENCES

Achenbach, T.M. and C. Edelbrock: 1991, Manual for the Youth Self-report and Profile (University of Vermont Department of Psychiatry, Burlington, VT).

Achenbach, T.M., S.H. McConaughy and C.T. Howell: 1987, 'Child/adolescent behavioral and emotional problems: Implications of cross-informant correlations for situational specificity', Psychological Bulletin 101, pp. 213–232.

Adelman, H.S., L. Taylor and P. Nelson: 1989, 'Minors' dissatisfaction with their life circumstances', Child Psychiatry and Human Development 20, pp. 135–147.

Andrews, F.M. and J.P. Robinson: 1991, 'Measures of subjective well-being', in J.P. Robinson, P.R. Shaver and L. Wrightsman (eds.), Social Psychological Attitudes: Vol. 1. Measures of Personality and Social Psychological Attitudes (Academic Press, San Diego, CA), pp. 61–114.

Andrews, F.M. and S.B. Withey: 1976, Social Indicators of Well-being: American's Perceptions of Life Quality (Plenum, New York).

Arnett, J.J.: 1999, 'Adolescent storm and stress, revisited', American Psychologist 54, pp. 371–386.

Ash, C. and Huebner, E.S.: 2002, 'Environmental events and life satisfaction reports of adolescents: A test of cognitive mediation', School Psychology International 22, pp. 320–336.

Bender, T.A.: 1997, 'Assessment of subjective well-being during childhood and adolescence', in G. Phye (ed.), Handbook of Classroom Assessment: Learning, Achievement, and Adjustment (Academic Press, San Diego, CA), pp. 199–225.

Brantley, A., E.S. Huebner and R. Nagle: 2002, 'Multidimensional life satisfaction reports of adolescents with mild mental disabilities', Mental Retardation 40, pp. 321–329.

Campbell, D., P. Converse and W. Rodgers: 1976, The Quality of American Life (Russell Sage Foundation, New York).

Casas, F., C. Alsinet, M. Rosich, E.S. Huebner and J.E. Laughlin: 2001, 'Cross-cultural investigation of the Multidimensional Students' Life Satisfaction Scale with Spanish adolescents', Paper presented at the Third Conference of the International Society for Quality of Life Studies, Girona, Spain.

Chamberlain, K.: 1988, 'On the structure of well-being', Social Indicators Research 20, pp. 581–604.

Compas, B.E., J. Conner and M. Wadsworth: 1997, 'Prevention of depression', in R.P. Weissberg, T.P. Gullotta, R.L. Hamptom, B.A. Ryan and G.R. Adams (eds.), Enhancing Children's Wellness (Sage, Thousand Oaks, CA), pp. 129–174.

Cowen, E.L.: 1991, 'In pursuit of wellness', American Psychologist 46, pp. 404–408.

Crenshaw, M.: 1998, 'Adjudicated violent youth, adjudicated non-violent youth vs. non-adjudicated, non-violent youth on selected psychological measures', Unpublished masters thesis, University of South Carolina.

Crocker, A.C.: 2000, 'Introduction: The happiness in all our lives', American Journal on Mental Retardation 105, pp. 319–325.

Cummins, R.A.: 2001, 'Personal income and subjective well-being: A review', Journal of Happiness Studies 1, pp. 133–158.

Cummins, R.A.: 1997, Manual for the Comprehensive Quality of Life Scale-Student (Grades 7–12): ComQol-S5, 5th edition (School of Psychology, Deakin University, Melbourne, Australia).

Day, H. and S.G. Jankey: 1996, 'Lessons from the literature: Toward a holistic model of quality of life', in R. Renwick, I. Brown and M. Nagler (eds.), Quality of Life in Health Promotion and Rehabilitation: Conceptual Approaches, Issues and Applications (Sage, Thousand Oaks, CA), pp. 39–50.

Dew, T.: 1996, 'The preliminary development and validation of a multidimensional life satisfaction scale for adolescents', Unpublished doctoral dissertation, University of South Carolina, Columbia.

Dew, T. and E.S. Huebner: 1994, 'Adolescents' perceived quality of life: An exploratory investigation', Journal of School Psychology 32, pp. 185–199.

Dew, T., E.S. Huebner and J.E. Laughlin: 2002, 'Preliminary development and validation of the Multidimensional Students' Life Satisfaction Scale B Adolescent version', Manuscript submitted for publication.

Diener, E.: 1994, 'Assessing subjective well-being: Progress and opportunities', Social Indicators Research 31, pp. 103–157.

Diener, E.: 1996, 'Traits can be powerful, but are not enough: Lessons from subjective well-being', Journal of Research in Personality 30, pp. 389–399.

Diener, E.: 2000, 'Subjective well-being: The science of happiness and a proposal for a national index', American Psychologist 55, pp. 34–43.

Diener, E. and Diener, M.: 1995, 'Cross-cultural correlates of life satisfaction and self-esteem', Journal of Personality and Social Psychology 68, pp. 653–663.

Diener, E. and Diener, C.: 1996, 'Most people are happy', Psychological Science 7, pp. 181–185.

Diener, E. and D.G. Myers: 1995, 'Who is happy?', Psychological Science 6, pp. 10–19.

Diener, E. and E. Suh: 1997, 'Measuring quality of life: Economic, social, and subjective indicators', Social Indicators Research 40, pp. 189–216.

Diener, E., R.A. Emmons, R.J. Larsen and S. Griffin: 1985, 'The Satisfaction With Life Scale', Journal of Personality Assessment 49, pp. 71–75.

Diener, E., E.M. Suh, R.E. Lucas and H.L. Smith: 1999, 'Subjective well-being: Three decades of progress', Psychological Bulletin 125, pp. 276–302.

Dryfoos, J.G.: 1990, Adolescents at Risk: Prevalence and Prevention (Oxford University Press, New York).

Elias, M.J.: 1989, 'Schools as a source of stress to children: An analysis of causal and ameliorative influences', Journal of School Psychology 27, pp. 393–407.

Evans, D.R.: 1994, 'Enhancing quality of life in the population at large', Social Indicators Research 33, pp. 47–88.

Farrell, A.D., R.F. Valois, A.L. Meyer and R. Tidwell: in press, 'Impact of the RIPP Violence Prevention Program on rural middle school students', Journal of Primary Prevention.

Felce, D. and J. Perry: 1996, 'Exploring current conceptions of quality of life: A model for people with and without disabilities', in R. Renwick, I. Brown and M. Nagler (eds.), Quality of Life in Health Promotion and Rehabilitation: Conceptual Approaches, Issues and Applications (Sage, Thousand Oaks, CA), pp. 39–50.

Fogle, L.M., E.S. Huebner and J.E. Laughlin: in press, 'The relationship between temperament and life satisfaction in adolescence: Cognitive and behavioral mediation models', Journal of Happiness Studies.

Frederickson, B.: 1998, 'What good are positive emotions?', Review of General Psychology 2, pp. 300–319.

Frisch, M.B.: 1998, 'Quality of Life Therapy and Assessment in health care', Clinical Psychology: Science and Practice 5, pp. 19–40.

Frisch, M.B., M.P. Clark, S.V. Rouse, M.P. Rudd, J. Paweleck, A. Greenstone and D. Kopplin: 2001, 'Predictive and treatment validity of the Quality of Life

Inventory in managed care, substance abuse, community mental health, and counseling center samples', Manuscript submitted for publication.
Frisch, M.B., J. Cornell, M. Villenueva and P.J. Retzlaff: 1992, 'Clinical validation of the Quality of Life Inventory: A measure of life satisfaction for use in treatment outcome assessment', Psychological Assessment 4, pp. 92–101.
Furr, R.M. and D. Funder: 1998, 'A multimodal analysis of personal negativity', Journal of Personality and Social Psychology 74, pp. 1580–1591.
Gilman, R.: 2001, 'The relationship between life satisfaction, social interest, and frequency of extracurricular activities among adolescent students', Journal of Youth and Adolescence 30, pp. 749–767.
Gilman, R. and M.L. Handwerk: 2001, 'Changes in life satisfaction as a function of stay in a residential setting', Residential Treatment for Children and Youth 18, pp. 47–65.
Gilman, R.S. and E.S. Huebner: 2000, 'Review of life satisfaction measures for adolescents', Behavior Change 17, pp. 178–195.
Gilman, R. and E.S. Huebner: 1997, 'Children's reports of their life satisfaction: Convergence across raters, time, and response formats', School Psychology International 18, pp. 229–243.
Gilman, R., E.S. Huebner and J.E. Laughlin: 2000, 'A first study of the Multidimensional Students' Life Satisfaction Scale with adolescents', Social Indicators Research 52, pp. 135–160.
Greene, A.L.: 1990, 'Patterns of affectivity in the transition to adolescence', Journal of Experimental Child Psychology 50, pp. 340–356.
Greenspoon, P.J. and D.H. Saklofske: 1997, 'Validity and reliability of the Multidimensional Students' Life Satisfaction Scale with Canadian children', Journal of Psychoeducational Assessment 15, pp. 138–155.
Greenspoon, P.J. and D.H. Saklofske: 2001, 'Toward an integration of subjective well-being and psychopathology', Social Indicators Research 54, pp. 81–108.
Griffin, M. and E.S. Huebner: 2000, 'Multidimensional life satisfaction reports of students with serious emotional disturbance', Journal of Psychoeducational Assessment 18, pp. 111–124.
Grob A., A. Stetsenko, C. Sabatier, L. Botcheva and P. Macek: 1999, 'A cross-national model of subjective well-being in adolescence', in F. Alsaker (ed.), The Adolescent Experience: European and American Adolescents in the 1990s (Erlbaum, Mahwah, NJ), pp. 115–130.
Gullone, E. and R.A. Cummins: 1999, 'The Comprehensive Quality of Life Scale: A psychometric evaluation with an adolescent sample', Behaviour Change 16, pp. 127–139.
Hammen, C. and K.P. Rudolph: 1996, 'Childhood depression', in F.J. Mash and R.A. Barkley (eds.), Child Psychopathology (Guildford, New York), pp. 153–195.
Headey, B., J. Kelly and A. Wearing: 1993, 'Dimensions of mental health: Life satisfaction, positive affect, anxiety, and depression', Social Indicators Research 29, pp. 63–82.

Heaven, P.C.: 1989, 'Extraversion, neuroticism, and satisfaction with life among adolescents', Personality and Individual Differences 10, pp. 489–492.
Hegarty, S.: 1994, 'Quality of life in school', in D. Goode (ed.), Quality of Life for Persons with Disabilities: International Perspectives and Issues (Brookline, Cambridge, MA), pp. 241–249.
Homel, R. and A. Burns: 1989, 'Environmental quality and the well-being of children', Social Indicators Research 21, pp. 133–158.
Huebner, E.S.: 1991a, 'Initial development of the Students' Life Satisfaction Scale', School Psychology International 12, pp. 231–240.
Huebner, E.S.: 1991b, 'Correlates of life satisfaction in children', School Psychology Quarterly 6, pp. 103–111.
Huebner, E.S.: 1991c, 'Further validation of the Students' Life Satisfaction Scale: The independence of satisfaction and affect ratings', Journal of Psychoeducational Assessment 9, pp. 363–368.
Huebner, E.S.: 1994a, 'Preliminary development and validation of a multidimensional life satisfaction scale for children', Psychological Assessment 6, pp. 149–158.
Huebner, E.S.: 1994b, 'Conjoint analyses of the Students' Life Satisfaction Scale and the Piers-Harris Self-Concept Scale', Psychology in the Schools 31, pp. 273–277.
Huebner, E.S.: 1995, 'The Students' Life Satisfaction Scale: An assessment of Psychometric properties with black and white elementary school students', Social Indicators Research 34, pp. 315–323.
Huebner, E.S.: 1997, 'Life satisfaction and happiness', In G. Bear, K. Minke and A. Thomas (eds.), Children's Needs II (National Association of School Psychologists, Silver Springs, MD), pp. 271–278.
Huebner E.S. and G.L. Alderman: 1993, 'Convergent and discriminant validation of a children's life satisfaction scale: Its relationship to self- and teacher-reported psychological problems and school functioning', Social Indicators Research 30, pp. 71–82.
Huebner, E.S., A. Brantley, R. Nagle and R. Valois: 2002, 'Correspondence between parent and adolescent ratings of life satisfaction for adolescents with and without mild mental disabilities', Journal of Psychoeducational Assessment 20, pp. 20–29.
Huebner, E.S. and T. Dew: 1993, 'An evaluation of racial bias in a life satisfaction scale', Psychology in the Schools 30, pp. 305–309.
Huebner, E.S. and T. Dew: 1996, 'The interrelationships of positive affect, negative affect, and life satisfaction in an adolescent sample', Social Indicators Research 38, pp. 129–137.
Huebner, E.S., W. Drane and R.F. Valois: 2000, 'Levels and demographic correlates of adolescent life satisfaction reports', School Psychology International 21, pp. 281–292.
Huebner, E.S., B.A. Funk and R. Gilman: 2000, 'Cross-sectional and longitudinal psychosocial correlates of adolescent life satisfaction reports', Canadian Journal of School Psychology 16, pp. 53–64.

Huebner, E.S., R. Gilman and J.E. Laughlin: 1999, 'A multimethod investigation of the multidimensionality of children's well-being reports: Discriminant validity of life satisfaction and self-esteem', Social Indicators Research 46, pp. 1–22.
Huebner, E.S., J.E. Laughlin, C. Ash and R. Gilman: 1998, 'Further validation of the Multidimensional Students' Life Satisfaction Scale', Journal of Psychoeducational Assessment 16, pp. 118–134.
Huebner, E.S. and G.C. McCullough: 2000, 'Correlates of school satisfaction among adolescents', Journal of Educational Research 93, pp. 331–335.
Kamman, R., M. Farry and P. Herbison: 1984, 'The analysis and measurement of happiness as a sense of well-being', Social Indicators Research 15, pp. 91–116.
Kazdin, A.: 1993, 'Adolescent mental health: Prevention and treatment programs', American Psychologist 48, pp. 127–141.
Landesman, S.: 1986, 'Quality of life and personal life satisfaction: Definition and measurement issues', Mental Retardation 91, pp. 141–143.
Laughlin, J.E. and E.S. Huebner: 2002, Unpublished data.
Lazarus, R.S.: 1991, Emotion and Adaptation (Oxford University Press, New York).
Lee, Y.T. and M.E.P. Seligman: 1997, 'Are Americans more optimistic than Chinese?' Personality and Social Psychology Prevention 23, pp. 32–40.
Leung, J. and K. Leung: 1992, 'Life satisfaction, self-concept, and relationship with parents in adolescence', Journal of Youth and Adolescence 21, pp. 653–665.
Lewinsohn, P., J. Redner and J. Seeley: 1991, 'The relationship between life satisfaction and psychosocial variables: New perspectives', in F. Strack, M. Argyle and N. Schwartz (eds.), Subjective Well-being (Plenum Press, New York), pp. 193–212.
Lucas, R.E., E. Diener and E. Suh: 1996, 'Discriminant validity of well-being measures', Journal of Personality and Social Psychology 71, pp. 616–628.
Man, P.: 1991, 'The influence of peers and parents on youth life satisfaction in Hong Kong', Social Indicators Research 24, pp. 347–365.
Maton, K.I.: 1990, 'Meaningful involvement instrumental activity and well-being. Studies of older adolescents and at risk urban teenagers', American Journal of Community Psychology 18, pp. 297–320.
McCullough, G., E.S. Huebner and J.E. Laughlin: 2000, 'Life events, self-concept, and adolescents' positive subjective well-being', Psychology in the Schools 37, pp. 281–290.
McCullough, M.E. and C.R. Snyder: 2000, 'Classical sources of human strength: Revisiting an old home and building a new one', Journal of Social and Clinical Psychology 19, pp. 1–10.
McKnight, C., E.S. Huebner and S.M. Suldo: 2002, 'Relationships among stressful life events, temperament, problem behavior, and global life satisfaction, Psychology in the Schools 39, pp. 677–687.
Neto, F.: 1993, 'The Satisfaction with Life Scale: Psychometric properties in an adolescent sample', Journal of Youth and Adolescence 22, pp. 125–134.

Newcomb, M.D., P.M. Bentler and C. Collins: 1986, 'Alcohol use and dissatisfaction with self and life: A longitudinal analysis of young adults', Journal of Drug Issues 63, pp. 479–494.

Park, N.: 2000, 'Life satisfaction among children and adolescents: Cross-cultural and cross-developmental comparisons', Unpublished doctoral dissertation, University of South Carolina.

Pavot, W. and E. Diener: 1993, 'Review of the Satisfaction With Life Scale', Psychological Assessment 5, pp. 164–172.

Petito, F. and R. Cummins: 2000, 'Quality of life in adolescents: The role of perceived control, parenting style, and social support', Behaviour Change 17, pp. 196–207.

Phillips, B.N.: 1993, Education and Psychological Perspectives on Stress in Students, Teachers and Parents (Clinical Psychology Publishing Company, Brandon, VT).

Piers, E.: 1984, Piers-Harris Children's Self-Concept Scale (Western Psychological Services, Los Angeles, CA).

Raphael, D., E. Rukholm, I. Brown, P. Hill-Bailey and E. Donato: 1996, 'The Quality of Life Profile-Adolescent Version: Background, description, and initial validation', Journal of Adolescent Health 19, pp. 366–375.

Reynolds, C.R. and R.W. Kamphaus: 1992, Manual for the Behavior Assessment System for Children (American Guidance Service, Inc, Circle Pines, MN).

Seligman, M.E.P.: 2002, Authentic Happiness (Free Press, New York).

Seligman, M.E.P. and M. Csikszentmihalyi: 2000, 'Positive psychology: An introduction', American Psychologist 55, pp. 5–14.

Seligson, J.L., E.S. Huebner and R.F. Valois: 2003, 'Preliminary validation of the Brief Multidimensional Student's Life Satisfaction Scale (BMSLSS)', Social Indicators Research 61, pp. 121–145.

Shek, D.T.: 1998, 'Adolescent positive mental health and psychological symptoms in a Chinese context', Psychologia 41, pp. 217–225.

Shin, D. and D.M. Johnson: 1978, 'Avowed happiness as an overall assessment of the quality of life', Social Indicators Research 5, pp. 475–492.

Smith, D.C., H.S. Adelman, P. Nelson, L. Taylor and V. Phares: 1987, 'Students' perceptions of control at school and problem behavior and attitudes', Journal of School Psychology 25, pp. 167–176.

Suldo, S.: 2001, 'Interrelationships among parenting behavior, life satisfaction, and adolescent behavior problems: A mediational model', Unpublished Masters thesis. University of South Carolina.

Suldo, S. and E.S. Huebner: in press. 'Does life satisfaction moderate the effects of stressful life events on psychopathological behavior in adolescence?' School Psychology Quarterly.

Terry, T. and E.S. Huebner: 1995, 'The relationship between self-concept and life satisfaction in children', Social Indicators Research 35, pp. 29–52.

Valois, R.E., K. Zullis, E.S. Huebner and W. Drane: 2001, 'Relationships between life satisfaction and violent behavior among adolescents', American Journal of Health Behavior 25, pp. 353–366.

Veenhoven, R.: 1988, 'The utility of happiness', Social Indicators Research 20, pp. 333–354.

Young, M.H., B.C. Miller, M.C. Norton and E.J. Hill: 1995, 'The effect of parental supportive behaviors on life satisfaction of adolescent offspring', Journal of Marriage and Family 57, pp. 813–822.

Zullig, K., R. Valois, E.S. Huebner and W. Drane: 2001, 'The relationship between life satisfaction and selected substance abuse behaviors among public high school adolescents', Journal of Adolescent Health 29, pp. 279–288.

Department of Psychology
University of South Carolina
Columbia, SC 29208
USA
E-mail: Huebner@sc.edu

AMANDA B. NICKERSON and RICHARD J. NAGLE

THE INFLUENCE OF PARENT AND PEER ATTACHMENTS ON LIFE SATISFACTION IN MIDDLE CHILDHOOD AND EARLY ADOLESCENCE

ABSTRACT. Satisfaction in different life domains was examined with respect to parent and peer attachment relationships in middle childhood and early adolescence. Three hundred three students, evenly distributed across sex and grade (fourth, sixth, and eighth) were administered *People in My Life*, a measure of attachment relationships, and the *Multidimensional Students' Life Satisfaction Scale*. Children and early adolescents in this sample generally reported high levels of life satisfaction. Some sex and grade differences in satisfaction with various life domains emerged. Attachments to both parents and peers predicted life satisfaction, although the influence of these relationships varied as a function of grade level and life domain. Findings are reviewed in relation to past research, and implications for professional practice are discussed.

KEY WORDS: attachment, early adolescence, life satisfaction, parents, peers

INTRODUCTION

The field of psychology is shifting its focus from examining deficits to building strengths (Seligman, 1999). This interest in primary prevention and competence building has been reflected in a blossoming body of research in psychological well-being and resilience in children (Cowen and Work, 1988; Diener, 1994; Doll and Lyon, 1998; Huebner, 1991a; Huebner and Dew, 1996). Subjective well-being is an individual's summary of the positive experiences in life, consisting of three components: global life satisfaction, positive affect, and negative affect. Life satisfaction is a person's evaluation of his or her life as a whole, which may be over and above judgments about family, friends, and school (Huebner, 1991a). Although this model of well-being was developed in reference to adults (Diener, 1994), it has been found to be applicable to children and adolescents aged eight and above (Huebner, 1997; Huebner and Dew, 1996).

Social Indicators Research **66:** 35–60, 2004.

Research on well-being has provided invaluable information about children's subjective judgments of their quality of life and has informed prevention and early intervention efforts. For instance, children consistently report high degrees of life satisfaction (Huebner, 1991b, 1997). Life satisfaction scores have generally been unrelated to age and sex (Huebner, 1991b, 1994, 1995, 1997), whereas personal predispositions, such as temperament, an internal locus of control, extraversion, and autonomy, are predictive of children's resilience and life satisfaction (Cowen and Work, 1988; Huebner, 1991a, 1997). Close relationships are also a major contributor to resilience and well-being, the most pronounced of these being the effects of a warm, supportive family environment, marked by a close relationship with at least one parent (Cotterell, 1992; Huebner, 1991a; Man, 1991; Paterson et al., 1994; Rice, 1990). Peer relationships and adult support systems outside the family are also correlated with resilience and life satisfaction (Cowen and Work, 1988; Doll and Lyon, 1998; Huebner, 1991a; Terry and Huebner, 1995).

Although close relationships are important for well-being, the large majority of studies investigating the influence of parent-child relationships have focused on maladaptive outcomes for children. Research on friendship has examined both positive and negative consequences, and has found that supportive friendships, particularly for girls, are positively correlated with school achievement, self-esteem, and psychosocial adjustment, and negatively correlated with school problems, loneliness, identity problems, and depression (Buhrmester, 1990; Bukowski et al., 1993; Hartup, 1996). Despite these empirical findings, there is no comprehensive developmental theory of friendship that attempts to explain its influence on children's social, emotional, and behavioral adjustment.

Attachment is a theoretically rich and empirically validated model for the study of the parent-child relationship, and it has been suggested that it serve as a model for all close relationships (Ainsworth, 1989; Hazan and Shaver, 1987, 1994). First described by Bowlby (1958), attachment behavior consists of proximity seeking, where the infant seeks closeness to the attachment figure, safe haven, where the infant seeks security in times of perceived danger or distress, and the secure base phenomenon, in which the infant explores his or her environment independent of the caregiver (Bretherton, 1985, 1992). It is believed that the attachment system is fully organized by the second year of life and that children construct complex internal working models, or mental representations, of the world, the persons in it, and the self (Bretherton, 1992).

Attachment relationships operate throughout the lifespan, although they change in form, becoming more reciprocal as individuals mature. Longitudinal studies have indicated that children with histories of secure attachment patterns are more competent, self-confident, and socially skilled than anxiously attached children (Elicker et al., 1992; Sroufe, 1989). Individual attachment patterns relate to peer and romantic relationships in adolescence, and attachment security is correlated with social competence and interpersonal functioning (Allen and Land, 1999; Rice, 1990). Similarly, older adolescents' and college students' security of attachment to parents is correlated with emotional functioning, social competence, a smoother balance of autonomy and attachment, and life satisfaction (Cotterell, 1992; Paterson et al., 1994; Rice, 1990). Adult attachment behavior is also linked to social functioning, with insecurely attached individuals having more interpersonal difficulties (Bartholomew, 1990, 1993; Crowell et al., 1999).

Despite the increasing use of attachment theory as a framework for the study of close relationships throughout the lifespan, two areas have been somewhat neglected in the literature. The first is the study of attachment relationships in middle childhood and early adolescence. Although attachment has been studied extensively in infancy, young childhood, and adulthood, the critical middle childhood and early adolescent years represent a gap in our knowledge. Second, although parent-child and romantic relationships have been examined within an attachment framework, the study of friendship has continued in the absence of a theoretical framework (Furman, 1993; Newcomb and Bagwell, 1995). Because friendships are such an integral part of early adolescence, using attachment as a theoretical framework for friendships is justified.

Early adolescence is a critical time for changes in parent and peer relationships. There is increased conflict in the parent-child relationship and early adolescents perceive their parents as less supportive

(Paikoff and Brooks-Gunn, 1991). In contrast, peers become a greater source of support (Allen and Land, 1999; Furman, 1989), loyalty and faithfulness in friendship become more critical (Berndt and Perry, 1990), and friends begin to compete less and share more equally (Berndt, 1989). One of the most salient features of early adolescent friendships is the support and intimacy that develops (Berndt and Perry, 1990; Lempers and Clark-Lempers, 1992). These features of friendship, such as trust and communication, are very similar to concepts in attachment theory.

When studying close relationships, it is crucial to consider the ways in which males and females differ. An oft-cited sex difference in friendship is that girls consistently report more intimacy and self-disclosure in their friendships, and this difference is most pronounced in early adolescence (Berndt and Perry, 1990; Buhrmester, 1990). Despite this consistent finding, sex differences have generally not been found in attachment research (Ainsworth, 1991; Hazan and Shaver, 1994), with the exception of a minority of studies with older adolescents finding that females scored higher than males on measures of peer attachment (Armsden and Greenberg, 1987; Paterson et al., 1994). Ainsworth (1991), a leader in the field of attachment, has suggested that sex differences and their manifestations in attachment relationships have yet to be discovered.

Statement of the Problem

Although research on the relationship between general social support and adjustment is plentiful, there is a need to study specific features of parent and close friendship relationships that contribute to life satisfaction (Berndt, 1989; Hartup, 1996; Huebner, 1991b). Given the success of attachment theory as a framework for the study of close relationships from infancy through adulthood, it is logical to apply this framework to investigations of early adolescents' relationships with parents and close friends, since friends have been shown to be so important to children at this age (Ainsworth, 1989; Furman, 1993; Hartup, 1996). In studying the manifestations of close relationships, there is a particular need to investigate developmental changes from childhood to adolescence and sex differences in close relationships and well-being.

The present study addressed these research needs by examining satisfaction with several life domains with respect to parent and peer attachment relationships in middle childhood and early adolescence. Sex differences in both life satisfaction and the influence of close relationships on life satisfaction were also explored. Specific questions included: (1) Does child and adolescent satisfaction with various life domains differ by grade and sex?, (2) Do parent and peer relationships predict satisfaction with various areas of life?, (3) Are there sex and/or grade differences in the relationship between parent and peer attachments and life satisfaction, (4) What specific aspects of children's relationships with parents and peers relate to their life satisfaction?

It was hypothesized that there would be no significant sex and grade differences for life satisfaction, as demographic variables have not consistently been correlated with this construct. Children's attachment relationships with parents were predicted to contribute the most variance in life satisfaction, especially for the domain of family life. It was also anticipated that attachment to peers would contribute to life satisfaction, and that this would correspond most strongly to satisfaction with friends. It was also hypothesized that the relationship between children's attachment to peers and their reports of life satisfaction would increase with age, so that the correlation for individuals in early adolescence would be higher than for those in middle childhood. Lastly, it was anticipated that trust in the parent and peer relationships would best predict life satisfaction.

METHOD

Subjects

Subjects consisted of 303 children from three elementary and three middle schools in a school district on the outskirts of a southeastern city. All students in these grades were given the opportunity to participate, but only those that returned parental permission were included in the study. There were 103 subjects in the fourth grade, 103 subjects in the sixth grade, and 97 subjects in the eighth grade. Children in the fourth grade were near the end of middle childhood, ranging from 8 to 11 years old, with a mean age of 9.61 ($SD = 0.57$); sixth grade students were in preadolescence, ranging from 11 to 14 years old, with a mean age of 11.67 ($SD = 0.71$); and eighth graders were in early adolescence, ranging in age from 13 to 15, with a mean age of 13.58 ($SD = 0.64$). Forty-eight percent of the sample was male and 52% was female, with 48 males and 55 females in the fourth grade, 49 males and 54 females in the sixth grade, and 47 males and 50 females in the eighth grade. Sixty-three percent of the sample was Caucasian, 32% was African-American, 1% was Hispanic/Latino, 2% was Asian, and 2% classified themselves as "Other".

Measures

People in My Life (Cook et al., 1995). *People in My Life*, a downward extension of Armsden and Greenberg's (1987) Inventory of Parent and Peer Attachment (IPPA), was used to assess children's attachments with parents and peers. Each item is rated on a 4-point scale from "Almost Never or Never True" (1 point) to "Almost Always or Always True" (4 points). The Parent Scale consists of 20 items, 10 of which assess Trust, five items that measure Communication, and five items that measure Alienation. The internal consistency coefficients for the present sample were $\alpha = 0.88$ (Parent Trust), $\alpha = 0.82$ (Parent Communication), and $\alpha = 0.70$ (Parent Alienation). The Peer Scale consists of 27 items, 10 of which assess Trust, five items that measure Communication, seven items that assess Alienation, and three items that measure Delinquency. The internal consistency coefficients for the present sample were $\alpha = 0.90$ (Peer Trust), $\alpha = 0.77$ (Peer Communication), $\alpha = 0.67$ (Peer Alienation), and $\alpha = 0.69$ (Peer Delinquency). Cook et al. (1995) conducted a preliminary study, showing that the reliability and validity of the Parent Scale and the Peer Scale of *People in My Life* were good.

Multidimensional Students' Life Satisfaction Scale (MSLSS; Huebner, 1994). Children's life satisfaction was assessed with the *MSLSS*, which assesses both global life satisfaction and satisfaction with specific life domains. This 40 item self-report scale consists of five subscales, which were derived from principal component analysis: School, Friends, Family, Self, and Living Environment. Each item is rated on a 4-point response scale: Never (1), Sometimes (2), Often (3), and Almost Always (4). The *MSLSS* shows adequate reliability and validity. The measurement quality of the scale is reported to be good (Greenspoon and Saklofske, 1997; Huebner et al., 1998). Internal consistency coefficients for the present sample were good, $\alpha = 0.83$ (School), $\alpha = 0.80$ (Friends), $\alpha = 0.84$ (Family), $\alpha = 0.77$ (Self), and $\alpha = 0.82$ (Living Environment). Test-retest reliability is adequate, ranging from 0.78 to 0.81 for the Total Scale and 0.53 to 0.81 for subscales over a four-week period (Greenspoon and Saklofske, 1997; Huebner et al., 1998). The convergent and discriminant validity of the *MSLSS* has been demonstrated by high correlations between almost every subscale and its targeted self-report criterion measure, and lower correlations with self-report nontargeted measures (Greenspoon and Saklofske, 1997; Huebner, 1994; Huebner et al., 1998).

Procedure

Students with parental consent to participate in the study were administered the *People in My Life* and *MSLSS* in groups ranging from approximately 10 to 25 students at their school. The measures were administered in counterbalanced order to each group of subjects. The researcher obtained student assent and asked them to complete a brief demographic information questionnaire. The researcher read the instructions and each item of the two measures for the fourth grade students, and read only the instructions for the sixth and eighth graders.

RESULTS

Grade and Sex Differences in Life Satisfaction

The mean response rating for Total Life Satisfaction, obtained by summing all 40 items and dividing by 40, was 3.09 (SD = 0.43), indicating that the sample had a moderately high level of overall satisfaction with life. There was some variation between the subscales of the *MSLSS*, ranging from a mean of 2.70 ($SD = 0.65$) for School Satisfaction to 3.35 ($SD = 0.52$) for Friends Satisfaction. To assess differences in life satisfaction as a function of sex and grade, a 2 (male vs. female) $\times$ 3 (fourth grade vs. sixth grade vs. eighth grade) *MANOVA* was conducted. There were significant sex

TABLE I

Means and standard deviations for MSLSS subscales by grade and sex

Scale	Grade			Sex	
	Fourth ($n = 103$)	Sixth ($n = 103$)	Eighth ($n = 97$)	Male ($n = 144$)	Female ($n = 159$)
Total satisfaction					
M	3.16	3.11	2.99	3.06	3.11
SD	0.43	0.41	0.44	0.41	0.45
Family satisfaction					
M	3.40	3.18	2.89	3.15	3.17
SD	0.50	0.61	0.65	0.60	0.65
Friends satisfaction					
M	3.37	3.35	3.35	3.33	3.38
SD	0.58	0.48	0.51	0.52	0.52
School satisfaction					
M	2.75	2.77	2.57	2.61	2.78
SD	0.72	0.62	0.59	0.56	0.71
Living environment satisfaction					
M	3.04	3.02	2.89	2.96	3.01
SD	0.67	0.61	0.61	0.64	0.63
Self satisfaction					
M	3.29	3.22	3.24	3.30	3.21
SD	0.59	0.53	0.53	0.51	0.58

differences, $F(5, 293) = 2.29$, $p < 0.05$ and grade differences, $F(10, 586) = 4.70$, $p < 0.001$, although the interaction between sex and grade was not significant.

As shown in Table I, females reported greater satisfaction with school than males, $F(1, 302) = 4.81$, $p < 0.05$, although there were no other significant sex differences. The only grade level difference was found for Family Satisfaction, $F(2, 301) = 18.74$, $p < 0.001$. As shown in Table I, fourth graders were most satisfied with their families, followed by sixth graders, with eighth graders reporting less satisfaction with families. Tukey's post hoc testing revealed that

TABLE II

Correlations of predictor and criterion variables for total sample

	1	2	3	4	5	6	7
1. Total satisfaction	—						
2. Family satisfaction	0.74**	—					
3. Friends satisfaction	0.71**	0.37**	—				
4. School satisfaction	0.70**	0.41**	0.28**	—			
5. Living satisfaction	0.82**	0.56**	0.48**	0.47**	—		
6. Self satisfaction	0.65**	0.39**	0.48**	0.28**	0.36**	—	
7. Parent attachment	0.60**	0.70**	0.32**	0.41**	0.48**	0.26**	—
8. Peer attachment	0.55**	0.32**	0.70**	0.31**	0.34**	0.38**	0.41**

Living satisfaction = Living environment satisfaction.
$^{**}p < 0.01$.

the differences between all three grade levels were significant, $p < 0.05$.

Relationships of Attachment and Life Satisfaction

To explore the relationship between children's attachments and life satisfaction, a series of multiple regression analyses were conducted. The correlations among the predictor variables (Parent and Peer Total Scales of *People in My Life*) and the criterion variables (Total Scale and subscales of the *MSLSS*) are displayed in Table II. Satisfaction with life in all domains was correlated significantly with parent attachment (r range = 0.26 to 0.70) and peer attachment (r range = 0.31 to 0.70).

As shown in Table III, the Parent and Peer Total Scales of *People in My Life* significantly predicted satisfaction with all life domains. Forty-seven percent of the variance in Total Life Satisfaction was explained by the model, and both parent and peer attachment contributed significantly. Although the model predicted 48% percent of the variance in Family Satisfaction, beta weights indicated that parent attachment, but not peer attachment, significantly contributed to the variance (see Table III). Similarly, although the regression model predicted 46% of the variance in Friends Satisfaction, beta weights indicated that peer attachment, but not parent

TABLE III

Regression models for effect of parent and peer attachment on satisfaction with life domains

Variable	β	t
Total life satisfaction		
Parent attachment	0.45	9.73**
Peer attachment	0.36	7.90**
	${R_{Adj}}^2 = 0.47$	$F(2, 300) = 132.75$**
Family satisfaction		
Parent attachment	0.68	15.01**
Peer attachment	0.04	0.783
	${R_{Adj}}^2 = 0.48$	$F(2, 300) = 141.95$**
Friends satisfaction		
Parent attachment	0.05	1.14
Peer attachment	0.66	14.16**
	${R_{Adj}}^2 = 0.46$	$F(2, 300) = 129.43$**
School satisfaction		
Parent attachment	0.34	5.93**
Peer attachment	0.17	2.90**
	${R_{Adj}}^2 = 0.18$	$F(2, 300) = 34.72$**
Living environment satisfaction		
Parent attachment	0.41	7.51**
Peer attachment	0.17	3.05**
	${R_{Adj}}^2 = 0.25$	$F(2, 300) = 50.99$**
Self satisfaction		
Parent attachment	0.12	2.09*
Peer attachment	0.33	5.66**
	${R_{Adj}}^2 = 0.15$	$F(2, 300) = 27.78$**

*$p < 0.05$; **$p < 0.001$.

attachment, significantly contributed to the variance. Parent and peer attachment significantly predicted School, Living Environment, and Self Satisfaction.

Sex and Grade Differences in Predictive Model

To assess for sex differences in predicting life satisfaction, the aforementioned multiple regression models were run separately for males and females. The results were consistent across sex for all models except for the prediction of School Satisfaction. Standardized regression coefficients indicated that both parent attachment ($\beta = 0.36$, $p < 0.001$) and peer attachment ($\beta = 0.17$, $p < 0.05$) significantly predicted School Satisfaction for females, but only parent attachment ($\beta = 0.33$, $p < 0.001$) predicted satisfaction with schools for males.

Grade differences were examined by conducting separate multiple regressions for fourth, sixth, and eighth graders. As shown in Table IV, there were grade differences in satisfaction with school, living environment, and self. Neither parent nor peer attachments predicted fourth graders' satisfaction with school, parent attachment, but not peer attachment, predicted sixth graders' satisfaction with school, and both parent and peer attachments predicted eighth graders' satisfaction with school. Only peer attachment predicted Living Environment Satisfaction for fourth graders, only parent attachment predicted satisfaction with living environment for sixth graders, and both parent and peer attachments predicted satisfaction with this domain of life for eighth graders. Self Satisfaction was predicted by peer attachment for students in each of the grades, although parent attachment significantly predicted Self Satisfaction for sixth graders only (see Table IV).

Dimensions of Attachment as Predictors of Life Satisfaction

To assess more specific effects of parent and peer attachment on life satisfaction, multiple regressions were conducted, using each of the subscales of *People in My Life* as predictor variables. As shown in Table V, all regression models were significant. The subscales of *People in My Life* significantly explained 51% of the variance in Total Life Satisfaction. All subscales of *People in My Life*, except for Parent Communication and Peer Communication, contributed

TABLE IV

Regression models for effect of parent and peer attachment on satisfaction with life domains by grade

Variable	Fourth graders		Sixth graders		Eighth graders	
	β	t	β	t	β	t
School satisfaction						
Parent attachment	0.06	0.52	0.49	5.40**	0.42	4.61**
Peer attachment	0.17	1.56	0.13	1.40	0.27	2.90*
	${R_{Adj}}^2 = 0.02$	$F(2, 100) = 2.12$	${R_{Adj}}^2 = 0.29$	$F(2, 100) = 21.70$**	${R_{Adj}}^2 = 0.33$	$F(2, 94) = 24.86$**
Living environment satisfaction						
Parent attachment	0.16	1.54	0.55	6.05**	0.48	5.44**
Peer attachment	0.26	2.55*	0.02	0.25	0.24	2.76*
	${R_{Adj}}^2 = 0.12$	$F(2, 100) = 7.60$**	${R_{Adj}}^2 = 0.29$	$F(2, 100) = 22.23$**	${R_{Adj}}^2 = 0.38$	$F(2, 94) = 30.20$**
Self satisfaction						
Parent attachment	–0.09	–0.84	0.30	3.07*	0.14	1.36
Peer attachment	0.43	4.19**	0.26	2.67*	0.31	2.99*
	${R_{Adj}}^2 = 0.16$	$F(2, 100) = 7.60$**	${R_{Adj}}^2 = 0.20$	$F(2, 100) = 13.46$**	${R_{Adj}}^2 = 0.14$	$F(2, 94) = 8.60$**

Only models with significant grade differences are reported.
$^{*}p < 0.01$; $^{**}p < 0.001$.

TABLE V

Regression models for effect of people in my life subscales on life satisfaction

Variable	β	t
Total life satisfaction		
Parent trust	0.34	4.88**
Parent communication	0.03	0.38
Parent alienation	–0.12	–2.51*
Peer trust	0.34	5.46**
Peer communication	0.01	0.16
Peer alienation	–0.11	–2.39*
Peer delinquency	–0.09	–2.14*
	${R_{Adj}}^2 = 0.51$	$F(7, 295) = 46.63$**
Family satisfaction		
Parent trust	0.52	7.88**
Parent communication	0.13	2.09*
Parent alienation	–0.10	–2.23*
Peer trust	0.08	1.40
Peer communication	–0.06	–1.09
Peer alienation	0.02	0.34
Peer delinquency	–0.16	–3.95**
	${R_{Adj}}^2 = 0.57$	$F(7, 295) = 57.25$**
Friends satisfaction		
Parent trust	–0.01	–0.12
Parent communication	–0.04	–0.60
Parent alienation	–0.05	–1.23
Peer trust	0.72	12.54**
Peer communication	–0.05	–1.02
Peer alienation	–0.17	–3.96**
Peer delinquency	0.03	0.77
	${R_{Adj}}^2 = 0.57$	$F(7, 295) = 58.79$**
School satisfaction		
Parent trust	0.17	1.88
Parent communication	0.08	0.96
Parent alienation	–0.09	–1.56
Peer trust	0.04	0.45

TABLE V

Continued

Variable	β	t
Peer communication	0.13	1.83
Peer alienation	–0.04	–0.60
Peer delinquency	–0.19	–3.34**
	$R_{Adj}^2 = 0.21$	$F(7, 295) = 12.12$**
Living environment satisfaction		
Parent trust	0.36	4.21**
Parent communication	–0.05	–0.61
Parent alienation	–0.17	–3.07**
Peer trust	0.12	1.60
Peer communication	–0.01	–0.16
Peer alienation	–0.12	–2.12*
Peer delinquency	–0.05	–0.97
	$R_{Adj}^2 = 0.28$	$F(7, 295) = 17.52$**
Self satisfaction		
Parent trust	0.20	2.23*
Parent communication	–0.03	–0.31
Parent alienation	0.04	0.59
Peer trust	0.32	3.96**
Peer communication	0.00	0.05
Peer alienation	–0.08	–1.39
Peer delinquency	0.06	1.10
	$R_{Adj}^2 = 0.18$	$F(7, 295) = 10.52$**

*$p < 0.05$; **$p < 0.001$.

significantly. The subscales of *People in My Life* explained 57% of the variance in Family Satisfaction. As shown in Table V, Parent Trust and Parent Communication contributed significantly to the variance in children's satisfaction with their families, as did Parent Alienation and Peer Delinquency, in a negative direction. The subscales of *People in My Life* explained 57% of the variance in Friends Satisfaction, with Peer Trust contributing the most variance to children's satisfaction with friends, followed by Peer Alienation, which contributed significantly in a negative direction.

The subscales of *People in My Life* predicted only 21% of the variance in School Satisfaction, and an examination of the beta weights indicates that only Peer Delinquency made a significant contribution, in an inverse direction. Twenty-eight percent of the variance in Living Environment Satisfaction was predicted by the regression model, with Parent Trust, Parent Alienation, and Peer Alienation making significant contributions (see Table V). The subscales of *People in My Life* predicted 18% of the variance in Self Satisfaction, and an examination of beta weights indicates that only the Parent and Peer Trust subscales contributed significantly.

DISCUSSION

The children and adolescents in this study reported moderately high degrees of life satisfaction, similar to the results of other studies of children and adolescents (Greenspoon and Saklofske, 1997; Huebner, 1991a, 1994, 1997). The majority of the sample reported being least satisfied with school, and most satisfied with friends, which is also consistent with past research (Greenspoon and Saklofske, 1997; Huebner, 1994).

There were few sex and grade differences in children's reports of life satisfaction. The trend of females reporting greater satisfaction with school than males has been found in previous studies with children (Huebner, 1994) and adolescents (Huebner et al., 2000). This finding is intriguing, given the ample literature documenting school-related difficulties for females in early adolescence, such as lower grades (Steinberg, 1993) and a decreased interest in certain subjects, such as mathematics and science (American Association of University Women, 1991). Boys report higher self-concepts in academics during elementary school, but report similar academic self-concepts to girls in high school (Wilgenbusch and Merrell, 1999). Therefore, it is possible that there is a shift during middle childhood and early adolescence, where boys become less comfortable with academics and less satisfied with school in general. Indeed, Pollack's (1998) work has highlighted similar evidence suggesting that boys' academic self-esteem suffers during early adolescence.

School satisfaction also differed by grade, with eighth graders reporting less satisfaction with school than sixth graders. This finding is consistent with numerous studies finding that adolescents in middle and junior high schools show a declining interest in school (Eccles et al., 1993; Montemayor and Flannery, 1990). Given that a significant proportion of high school students are dissatisfied with school (Huebner et al., 2000), and that dissatisfaction with school is the most common reason given by students for dropping out (U.S. Department of Education, 1990), the identification of eighth grade as a possible starting point for this trend has particular relevance for prevention efforts.

The only other grade difference found was for satisfaction with families, which decreased significantly as grade increased. It is reasonable to infer that, as adolescents begin to communicate less with their parents and feel as though their parents do not understand them, overall satisfaction with their families decreases. Of course, the relationship between these variables is likely bi-directional, whereby decreased satisfaction with families may lead to impaired communication with parents.

The overall picture that emerges regarding life satisfaction is that adolescents, compared to younger children, are less satisfied with their schools and families. Previous research regarding the stability of this trend, and its implications, is conflicting. Demographic variables have generally not been correlated, or have only related weakly to life satisfaction (Huebner, 1991a, 1995, 1997). However, some studies have found life satisfaction for individuals in mid-adolescence to be relatively low, especially in comparison to early adolescence (Man, 1991) and adulthood (Petito and Cummins, 2000). If adolescence does, indeed, represent a time of decreased satisfaction with life, the causes and implications of this are still speculative. For example, it is possible that adolescents' development of critical thinking skills leads them to be more critical and discerning when assessing and reporting their satisfaction with various aspects of life (Man, 1991). Alternatively, the increasing autonomy of adolescence may cause a problem of fit between their needs and the constraints of family and school (see e.g., Eccles et al., 1993; Montemayor and Flannery, 1990), resulting in genuine unhappiness with their present situation. Recent research has suggested that, even though increased conflict with parents is present in early adolescence, this conflict does not have long-lasting effects on the closeness of the parent-child relationship (Arnett, 1999). This important issue warrants further investigation, so that the nature of this dissatisfaction with life, and its implications, can be explored in greater depth.

Attachment relationships, either with parents, peers, or both, predicted satisfaction with all domains of life for the children and adolescents in this study. As anticipated, positive aspects of the parent and peer relationships, such as trust and communication, were highly correlated with children's overall life satisfaction. In addition, alienation from parents and peers was negatively correlated with life satisfaction, as was peer delinquency. Analyses of the contribution of parent and peer attachment to satisfaction with each domain of life yielded more specific information. Because the sample was not random, p-values were interpreted with extreme caution and priority was given to the size of estimates.

Parent trust was the best predictor of satisfaction with families. Communication with parents also predicted satisfaction, and alienation from parents was inversely related to family satisfaction. These findings are supported by attachment theory, which suggests that security, open communication, and understanding in the parent-child relationship is related to positive outcomes (Man, 1991; Paterson et al., 1994).

Peer delinquency, assessed by children's reports of their peers' influence on truancy, cheating, and drinking alcohol, was also inversely related to satisfaction with families. Research has confirmed that delinquent behavior in early adolescence is related to several family variables, such as lack of parental monitoring (Vazsonyi and Flannery, 1997), communication problems (Clark and Shields, 1997), and insecure parent-child attachments (Cashwell and Vacc, 1996; Vazsonyi and Flannery, 1997).

Peer trust was found to be the best predictor of satisfaction with friends. This finding validates the importance of commitment between friends, such as mutual caring, mutual liking, and trust/loyalty (Hartup, 1989; Newcomb and Bagwell, 1995). Peer communication and satisfaction with friends were significantly correlated. However, once the Parent Trust subscale was entered into the regression analysis, the Peer Communication subscale did not add unique variance to Friends Satisfaction. Because of their strong correlation, peer communication should not be regarded as unimportant to children's satisfaction with their friends, especially in light of past research indicating that verbal disclosure and intimacy are of central importance at this developmental period (Berndt and Perry, 1990; Lempers and Clark-Lempers, 1992).

Peer alienation also contributed significantly to satisfaction with friends, in an inverse direction. Previous research has shown that peer rejection and loneliness are linked to maladaptive outcomes for children (McFadyen-Ketchum and Dodge, 1998), although this has been studied less in adolescence. This indicates that alienation from peers continues to be a problem in middle childhood through early adolescence, as evidenced by its effect on this aspect of life satisfaction.

Peer delinquency was the only variable that significantly predicted satisfaction with school. There is a strong negative relationship between school variables (e.g., achievement, commitment to education) and delinquent behaviors (Vazsonyi and Flannery, 1997), and adolescents who are involved in structured extracurricular activities are less likely to exhibit deviant behaviors (Mahoney and Stattin, 2000). These school variables likely relate to school satisfaction, making peer delinquency incompatible with school satisfaction.

The effect of parent and peer attachments on school satisfaction differed by sex and grade. Peer attachments predicted school satisfaction for females but not for males. Cotterell (1992) found that girls' academic adjustment was related to support from parents and teachers, whereas boys' academic adjustment was not related to support from these adults, and was actually inversely related to support from friends. Perhaps peers have a differential impact on school satisfaction for males and females, with peers having a minimal, or even negative influence on boys' school satisfaction and academic adjustment. This difference may reflect values of males and females in contemporary society, where males, on average, spend more time in non-academic related activities (e.g., sports, watching television) and females spend more time studying and reading for pleasure (Halpern, 1997). Thus, boys and their close friends may value and find satisfaction in recreational activities rather than school.

Both peer and parent attachments failed to predict school satisfaction for fourth graders and only parent attachment predicted satisfaction for sixth graders. However, both parent and peer attachments predicted school satisfaction for eighth graders. This suggests that as children progress in school, peers take on increasing importance while parental influences continue to be important in shaping school satisfaction. It is possible that for fourth graders, such variables as teacher characteristics or school climate contribute their satisfaction with school. Indeed, a recent study found the teacher-student relationship to be a necessary condition for students' school satisfaction and engagement in academics (Rosenfield et al., 2000).

Satisfaction with living environment was predicted by both parent and peer attachments. The Living Environment Satisfaction subscale of the *MSLSS* consists of a broad range of items assessing satisfaction with the child's home, neighborhood, and people in the community and it is logical that both parent and peer attachments predict satisfaction with this area of life. Parent trust was a significant predictor, suggesting that children's security in their relationship with parents was central to their liking where they live. Parent and peer alienation also contributed significantly to living environment satisfaction, in an inverse direction. This is consistent with past research, which has found alienation from peers affects children's happiness (Homel and Burns, 1989).

Living environment satisfaction was also found to vary by grade level. Parent attachment did not predict satisfaction for fourth graders, and peer attachment failed to predict satisfaction for sixth graders. This pattern of results is difficult to explain although it may be speculated that subjects may have varied in their interpretations of the items regarding Living Environment Satisfaction on the *MSLSS*. Because this subscale assesses many areas of the living environment, such as the child's home, neighborhood, and more general community, children may appraise the items very differently. As a result, it is possible that fourth graders thought more about physical aspects of their home and neighborhoods when answering the questions, whereas sixth graders may have focused more on their home and family life within the neighborhood. Eighth graders, with their increasing complex thinking skills (Montemayor and Flannery, 1990; Vernon and Al-Mabuk, 1995), may have been able to more fully integrate different aspects of their living environment, such as physical and interpersonal characteristics of their homes, personal qualities of neighbors, including their peers, and facets of their community, such as social cohesiveness and safety.

Both parent and peer attachments predicted satisfaction with self. Peer trust was a significant contributor to self satisfaction across both sexes and all grades. Parent trust also predicted satisfaction with the self, except for sixth graders. Perhaps as early adolescents navigate the transition to middle school, parents become less important or their behavior is more highly scrutinized, at least temporarily. Evidence for the transient nature of parents' lack of importance in self satisfaction comes not only from this study's findings that parents are important for eighth graders' satisfaction, but also from studies showing parents to be central to self-esteem for middle and high school students (Rosenfeld et al., 2000).

Collectively, satisfaction with various aspects of life was predicted by parent and peer attachment relationships. Findings varied as a function of domain of life being studied, lending support to the notion that preadolescents can differentiate among specific domains in their lives (Huebner, 1994), and that multidimensional assessment models provide a rich picture of this phenomenon (Huebner et al., 1998). Across domains, parent and peer trust were particularly important predictor variables, suggesting that loyalty, trust, and commitment in these relationships contribute to life satisfaction for children and adolescents. Alienation, especially from peers, was also a salient predictor of dissatisfaction with school and living environment, implying that peer rejection and loneliness may be threats to well-being at this age. Finally, peer delinquency was inversely related to satisfaction both with families and school, which was consistent with delinquency literature positing a relationship between family process variables, school interest and achievement, and deviant behavior (Vazsonyi and Flannery, 1997).

A difficulty in conducting research on attachments for children in this age group is the lack of appropriate measures. Although *People in My Life* was the best instrument available, there are some notable limitations of this assessment tool. First, it assesses various aspects of attachment to parents and peers, in general, as opposed to asking about individual friends. Therefore, asking children and early adolescents to rate their attachments to peers, as opposed to a friend with whom they have a close relationship, may not accurately assess the attachment relationship. Second, the questions about parents and peers on *People in My Life* are very similar. Given that attachment to peers is theorized to be different from the parent-child attachment relationship, it would follow that procedures for assessing attachment between friends would be different. Another limitation of this instrument is the lack of research on its psychometric properties. The future development and validation of psychometrically sound measures of attachment for adolescents will be needed to further study the role of attachment in life satisfaction.

The current findings also suggest that the transition from middle childhood to early adolescence is critical in negotiating close relationships. Upon entry into early adolescence, peers become central sources of companionship and emotional support. Close peer relationships relate to various aspects of life satisfaction, suggesting that the development of these relationships should be encouraged. Schools are ideal settings in which to promote resiliency and competency in children (Doll and Lyon, 1998), and efforts should be made to facilitate the development of close peer relationships.

Boys' decreased satisfaction with school also has implications for professional practice. Given that school satisfaction is related to the likelihood of students remaining in school (Ainley et al., 1991), it is critical for school personnel to make efforts to engage boys in school. Due, in part, to the widely published surveys citing American schools' shortchanging of girls (e.g., American Association of University Women, 1991), schools have been sensitized to the needs of girls. However, findings from this study indicate that boys are more dissatisfied with school than girls. In addition, males consistently receive lower grades in school than females and are over-represented in the low-ability end of several learning and cognitive disability distributions (Halpern, 1997). They are also somewhat more likely to drop out of school (Ainley et al., 1991; Kaufman et al., 1999). Taken together, these findings suggest that schools need to proceed cautiously to ensure that they are not shortchanging boys in their quest to be sensitive to issues facing girls (Pollack, 1998).

Peer alienation and delinquency proved to be central to several aspects of life satisfaction, indicating that prevention and intervention efforts should target children who are lonely, alienated from peers, and involved in deviant behavior. In a time when treatment too often focuses on externalizing behaviors, these results indicate that peer rejection and loneliness should also be addressed due to their far-reaching implications.

REFERENCES

Ainley, J., J. Foreman and M. Sheret: 1991, 'High school factors that influence students to remain in school', Journal of Educational Research 85, pp. 69–80.

Ainsworth, M.D.S.: 1989, 'Attachments beyond infancy', American Psychologist 44, pp. 709–716.

Ainsworth, M.D.S.: 1991, 'Attachments and other affectional bonds across the life cycle', in C.M. Parkes, J. Stevenson-Hinde and P. Marris (eds.), Attachment Across the Life Cycle (Tavistock/Routledge, New York), pp. 33–51.

Allen, J.P. and D. Land: 1999, 'Attachment in adolescence', in J. Cassidy and P.R. Shaver (eds.), Handbook of Attachment: Theory, Research, and Clinical Applications (Guilford, New York), pp. 319–335.

American Association of University Women: 1991, Shortchanging Girls, Shortchanging America: Executive Summary (American Association of University Women, Washington DC).

Armsden, G.C. and M.T. Greenberg: 1987, 'The inventory of parent and peer attachment: Individual differences and their relationships to psychological well-being in adolescence', Journal of Youth and Adolescence 16, pp. 427–454.

Arnett, J.J.: 1999, 'Adolescent storm and stress, reconsidered', American Psychologist 54, pp. 317–326.

Bartholomew, K.: 1990, 'Avoidance of intimacy: An attachment perspective', Journal of Social and Personal Relationships 7, pp. 147–178.

Bartholomew, K.: 1993, 'From childhood to adult relationships: Attachment theory and Research', in S. Duck (ed.), Learning About Relationships (Sage, Newbury Park, CA), pp. 30–62.

Berndt, T.J.: 1989, 'Obtaining support from friends during childhood and adolescence', in D. Belle (ed.), Children's Social Networks and Social Support (John Wiley and Sons, New York), pp. 308–331.

Berndt, T.J. and T.B. Perry: 1990, 'Distinctive feature and effects of early adolescent Friendships', in R. Montemayor, G.R. Adams and T.P. Gullotta (eds.), From Childhood to Adolescence: A Transitional Period? (Sage, Newbury Park, CA), pp. 269–287.

Bowlby, J.: 1958, 'The nature of the child's tie to his mother', International Journal of Psychoanalysis 35, pp. 350–373.
Bretherton, I.: 1985, 'Attachment theory: Retrospect and prospect', in I. Bretherton and E. Waters (eds.), Growing Points of Attachment Theory and Research, Monographs of the Society for Research in Child Development 50, pp. 3–35.
Bretherton, I.: 1992, 'The origins of attachment theory: John Bowlby and Mary Ainsworth', Developmental Psychology 28, pp. 759–775.
Buhrmester, D.: 1990, 'Intimacy of friendship, interpersonal competence, and adjustment during middle childhood and adolescence', Child Development 61, pp. 1101–1111.
Bukowski, W.M., B. Hoza and M. Boivin: 1993, 'Popularity, friendship, and emotional adjustment during early adolescence', in W. Damon (series ed.) and B. Laurson (vol. ed.), New Directions for Child Development: Vol. 60. Close Friendships in Adolescence (Jossey-Bass, San Francisco, CA), pp. 23–37.
Cashwell, C.S. and N.A. Vacc: 1996, 'Family functioning and risk behaviors: Influences on adolescent delinquency', School Counselor 44, pp. 105–114.
Clark, R.D. and G. Shields: 1997, 'Family communication and delinquency', Adolescence 32, pp. 81–92.
Cook, E.T., M.T. Greenberg and C.A. Kusche: 1995, 'People in My Life: Attachment relationships in middle childhood', poster presented at the Society for Research in Child Development (Indianapolis, IN).
Cotterell, J.L.: 1992, 'The relation of attachments and support to adolescent well-being and school adjustment', Journal of Adolescent Research 7, pp. 28–42.
Cowen, E.L. and W.C. Work: 1988, 'Resilient children, psychological wellness, and primary Prevention', American Journal of Community Psychology 16, pp. 591–607.
Crowell, J.A., R.C. Fraley and P.R. Shaver: 1999, 'Measurement of individual differences in adolescent and adult attachment', in J. Cassidy and P.R. Shaver (eds.), Handbook of Attachment: Theory, Research, and Clinical applications (Guilford, New York), pp. 434–465.
Diener, E.: 1994, 'Assessing subjective well-being: Progress and opportunities', Social Indicators Research 31, pp. 103–157.
Doll, B. and M.A. Lyon: 1998, 'Risk and resilience: Implications for the delivery of educational and mental health services in schools', School Psychology Review 27, pp. 348–363.
Eccles, J.S., C. Midgley, A. Wigfield, R.M. Buchanan, D. Reuman, C. Flanagan and D. MacIver: 1993, 'Development during adolescence: The impact of stage-environment fit on young adolescents' experiences in schools and families', American Psychologist 48, pp. 90–101.
Elicker, J., M. Englund and L.A. Sroufe: 1992, 'Predicting peer competence and peer relationships in childhood from early parent-child relationships', in R.D. Parke and G.W. Ladd (eds.), Family-Peer Relationships: Modes of Linkage (Lawrence Erlbaum, Hillsdale, NJ), pp. 77–106.

Furman, W.: 1989, 'The development of children's social networks', in D. Belle (ed.), Children's Social Networks and Social Support (John Wiley and Sons, New York), pp. 151–172.
Furman, W.: 1993, 'Theory is not a four-letter word: Needed directions in the study of adolescent friendships', in B. Laursen (ed.), Close Friendships in Adolescence: New Directions for Child Development, 60 (Jossey-Bass, San Francisco, CA), pp. 89–103.
Greenspoon, P.J. and D.H. Saklofske: 1997, 'Validity and reliability of the multidimensional students' life satisfaction scale with Canadian children', Journal of Psychoeducational Assessment 15, pp. 138–155.
Halpern, D.F.: 1997, 'Sex differences in intelligence: Implications for education', American Psychologist 52, pp. 1091–1102.
Hartup, W.W.: 1989, 'Social relationships and their developmental significance', American Psychologist 44, pp. 120–126.
Hartup, W.W.: 1996, 'The company they keep: Friendships and their developmental significance', Child Development 67, pp. 1–13.
Hazan, C. and P.R. Shaver: 1987, 'Romantic love conceptualized as an attachment process', Journal of Personality and Social Psychology 52, pp. 511–524.
Hazan, C. and P.R. Shaver: 1994, 'Attachment as an organizational framework for research on close relationships', Psychological Inquiry 5, pp. 1–22.
Homel, R. and A. Burns: 1989, 'Environmental quality and the wellbeing of children', Social Indicators Research 21, pp. 133–158.
Huebner, E.S.: 1991a, 'Correlates of life satisfaction in children', School Psychology Quarterly 6, pp. 103–111.
Huebner, E.S.: 1991b, 'Initial development of the Student's Life Satisfaction Scale', School Psychology International 12, pp. 231–240.
Huebner, E.S.: 1994, 'Preliminary development and validation of a multidimensional life satisfaction scale for children', Psychological Assessment 6, pp. 149–158.
Huebner, E.S.: 1995, 'The students' life satisfaction scale: An assessment of psychometric properties with black and white elementary school students', Social Indicators Research 34, pp. 315–323.
Huebner, E.S.: 1997, 'Life satisfaction and happiness', in G.G. Bear, K.M. Minke and A. Thomas (eds.), Children's Needs II: Development, Problems, and Alternatives (National Association of School Psychologists, Bethesda, MD), pp. 271–278.
Huebner, E.S. and T. Dew: 1996, 'The interrelationship of positive affect, negative affect, and life satisfaction in an adolescent sample', Social Indicators Research 38, pp. 129–137.
Huebner, E.S., W. Drane and R.F. Valois: 2000, 'Levels and demographic correlates of adolescent life satisfaction reports', School Psychology International 21, pp. 281–292.
Huebner, E.S., J.E. Laughlin, C. Ash and R. Gilman: 1998, Further validation of the Multidimensional Students' Life Satisfaction Scale', Journal of Psychoeducational Assessment 16, pp. 118–134.

Kaufman, P., S. Klein and M. Frase: 1999, Dropout Rates in the United States: 1997 (U.S. Department of Education, Washington, DC).
Lempers, J.D. and D.S. Clark-Lempers: 1992, 'Young, middle, and late adolescents' comparisons of the functional importance of five significant relationships', Journal of Youth and Adolescence 21, pp. 53–96.
Mahoney, J.L. and H. Stattin: 2000, 'Leisure activities and adolescent antisocial behavior: The role of structure and social context', Journal of Adolescence 23, pp. 113–127.
Man, P.: 1991, 'The influence of peers and parents on youth life satisfaction in Hong Kong', Social Indicators Research 24, pp. 347–365.
McFadyen-Ketchum, S. A. and K.A. Dodge: 1998, 'Problems in social relationships', in E.J. Mash and R.A. Barkley (eds.), Treatment of Childhood Disorders: Second Edition (Guilford, New York), pp. 338–365.
Montemayor, R. and D.J. Flannery: 1990, 'Making the transition from childhood to early adolescence', in R. Montemayor, G.R. Adams and T.P. Gullotta (eds.), From Childhood to Adolescence: A Transitional Period? (Sage, Newbury Park, CA), pp. 269–287.
Newcomb, A.F. and C.L. Bagwell: 1995, 'Children's friendship relations: A meta-analytic review', Psychological Bulletin 117, pp. 306–347.
Paikoff, R.L. and J. Brooks-Gunn: 1991, 'Do parent-child relationships change during puberty?', Psychological Bulletin 110, pp. 47–66.
Paterson, J.E., J. Field and J. Pryor: 1994, 'Adolescents' perceptions of their attachment relationships with their mothers, fathers, and friends', Journal of Youth and Adolescence 23, pp. 579–600.
Petito, F. and R.A. Cummins: 2000, 'Quality of life in adolescence: The role of perceived control, parenting style, and social support', Behaviour Change 17, pp. 196–207.
Pollack, W.: 1998, Real Boys: Rescuing our Sons From the Myths of Boyhood (Henry Holt, New York).
Rice, K.G.: 1990, 'Attachment in adolescence: A narrative and meta-analytic review', Journal of Youth and Adolescence 19, pp. 511–538.
Rosenfield, L.B., J.M. Richman and G.L. Bowen: 2000, 'Social support networks and school outcomes: The centrality of the teacher', Child and Adolescent Social Work Journal 17, pp. 205–226.
Seligman, M.E.P.: 1999, 'Teaching positive psychology', APA Monitor, p. 42.
Sroufe, L.A.: 1989, 'Pathways to adaptation and maladaptation: Psychopathology as developmental deviation', in D. Cicchetti (ed.), The Emergence of a Discipline: Rochester Symposium on Developmental Psychopathology, Vol. 1 (Lawrence Erlbaum, Hillsdale, NJ), pp. 13–40.
Steinberg, A.: 1993, Adolescents and Schools: Improving the Fit (Harvard University, Cambridge, MA).
Terry, T. and E.S. Huebner: 1995, 'The relationship between self-concept and life satisfaction in children', Social Indicators Research 35, pp. 39–52.

U.S. Department of Education: 1990, National Center for Education Statistics, National Education Longitudinal Study of 1988: First Followup Study, 1990 (U.S. Department of Education, Washington, DC).
Vazsonyi, A.T. and D.J. Flannery: 1997, 'Early adolescent delinquent behaviors: Associations with family and school domains', Journal of Early Adolescence 17, pp. 271–293.
Vernon, A. and R.H Al-Mabuk: 1995, What Growing Up is All About: A Parent's Guide to Child and Adolescent Development (Research Press, Champaign, IL).
Wilgenbusch, T. and K.W. Merrell: 1999, 'Gender differences in self-concept among children and adolescents: A meta-analysis of multidimensional studies', School Psychology Quarterly 14, pp. 101–120.

Department of Educational and Counseling Psychology
ED 232
University at Albany – State University of New York
Albany, NY 12222
USA
E-mail: anickerson@uamail.albany.edu

NANSOOK PARK, E. SCOTT HUEBNER, JAMES E. LAUGHLIN,
ROBERT F. VALOIS and RICH GILMAN

A CROSS-CULTURAL COMPARISON OF THE DIMENSIONS OF CHILD AND ADOLESCENT LIFE SATISFACTION REPORTS

ABSTRACT. The factorial invariance of the Multidimensional Students' Life Satisfaction Scale (MSLSS: Huebner, 1994) across two divergent cultures (collectivistic vs. individualistic) was investigated with 835 Korean and 822 US students in elementary, middle, and high schools. Psychometric properties of the Korean version of the MSLSS were acceptable. A series of multisample-confirmatory factor analyses (MCFA) demonstrated the cross-cultural similarity of the five-factor model for students' life satisfaction. The similar structure of MSLSS across cultural groups provides the basis for meaningful international comparisons of life satisfaction among children and adolescents. Further cross-cultural research including various culturally sensitive life satisfaction domains may enhance understanding of cultural differences in the structure, correlates, and consequences related to students' life satisfaction.

The psychological importance of subjective well-being (SWB) on the overall quality of social and personal life of individuals has increasingly been recognized (Strack et al., 1991). Life satisfaction, a person's cognitive appraisal of the quality of his or her life circumstance, is one aspect of positive SWB (Diener and Diener, 1995; Shin and Johnson, 1978; Veenhoven, 1996). Research has demonstrated that individuals with lower life satisfaction are at risk for a variety of psychological and social problems such as depression, low self-esteem, and maladaptive social interactions (Furr and Funder,1998; Lewinsohn et al., 1991).

Although numerous studies have been done with adults, researchers have only recently begun to examine the structure of life satisfaction in children and adolescents. Furthermore, most of the research concerning children's life satisfaction has used unidimensional measures, which have offered limited information regarding the underlying structure of life satisfaction in children and adolescents. One exception is the Multidimensional Students' Life

Social Indicators Research **66:** 61–79, 2004.

Satisfaction Scale (MSLSS: Huebner, 1994), which is designed to measure children's subjective perceptions of life satisfaction in five relevant domains: Family, Friends, School, Living Environment, and Self as well as overall life satisfaction.

Studies of the construct validity of the MSLSS with American students using exploratory and confirmatory factor analysis have supported the proposed five-factor model (Gilman et al., 2000; Huebner et al., 1998). However, there are only a few studies which examined the psychometric properties (e.g., the generalizability of the factor structure) of the MSLSS in other cultures. The results of a study with a large sample of Canadian children in grades 3 to 8 (Greenspoon and Saklofske, 1997) and a study with students from Spain in grade 9 to 11 using a Catalan version of the MSLSS (Casas et al., 2001) reported adequate internal consistency and supported the five-factor structure of the scale. Although research to date with the MSLSS has demonstrated good psychometric properties and a consistent five-factor structure, the research has been limited mostly to samples from Western, individualistic cultures with a limited age range.

Frequent concerns have been expressed regarding the cross-cultural comparability of psychological measurements. Increasing numbers of research studies have demonstrated that cultural experiences influence an individual's social, emotional, and cognitive development (Basic Behavioral Science Task Force, 1996). For example, cross-cultural studies reported that in collectivistic Eastern cultures, where the harmony with members of important groups (e.g., family, schools) is highly valued, individual's psychological processes are influenced by others' perspectives and societal norms (Markus and Kitayama, 1991, 1994). In contrast, in individualistic cultures such as those in North America, where the self is regarded as an independent entity, personal interests and inner feelings tend to be valued more and are primary sources in the life satisfaction judgment process (Suh et al., 1998). Thus, these cultural differences may influence on individual's interpretation and responses to items measuring life satisfaction (Riordan and Vandenberg, 1994).

With respect to measurement issues in comparative cross-cultural studies, Bond and Task-sking (1983) argued that many of the cross-cultural studies of psychological constructs have used instruments developed on American samples with individuals in non-Western cultures. Researchers have then compared American and non-Western individuals without considering the psychometric comparability of the instruments. Lack of equivalence in validity of the instruments may suggest differences in the meaning of life satisfaction constructs in different cultural groups.

Measurement equivalence means that items on the scale are interpreted and responded to in the same way across groups (Little, 2000). Construct comparability (factor invariance) holds when the corresponding measurement parameters (factor loadings) of a construct are equivalent across groups of interest (Meredith, 1993). When this condition has been met, then the cultural differences in levels, correlates, and consequences related to constructs can be examined in valid and meaningful ways (Little, 2000). For example, although some researchers have explored mean differences in life satisfaction across culturally diverse groups (e.g., Diener and Diener, 1995; Huebner, 1998; Man, 1991; Suh et al., 1998), the methodological focus on the extent to which life satisfaction measures are equivalent across cultures has often been overlooked (Byrne, 1996). If measures cannot be shown to be equivalent across the groups of interest, then any comparisons of mean differences will be meaningless. Similarly, comparisons of correlates and consequences related to the construct will be questionable. Thus, it is imperative that the researchers assess the construct validity of measuring instruments with diverse cultural groups before investigating differential levels of well-being.

Considering research findings on possible differences in life satisfaction between individualistic and collectivistic cultures (e.g., Diener and Diener, 1995), research investigating the reliability and construct validity of the MSLSS with students from non-Western cultures, such as Korea, should be conducted as part of instrument development. The purpose of current study was to investigate the comparability of the factor structure of the MSLSS (Huebner, 1994) between Korean and American students of three age levels (elementary, middle, and secondary school age).

Previous studies using the MSLSS with American students reported five related but separable factors corresponding to each of the five domains of the MSLSS (Family, Friends, School,

Self, Living Environment) (Huebner, 1994; Huebner et al., 1998). However, due to the collectivistic nature of the Korean culture, which is different from the individualistic American culture (Suh et al., 1998), the Self domain of the MSLSS may not be separable from other domains. Koreans think of themselves using more group-related concepts than do Americans and thus see their ideal "self" as being closer to their social self than Westerners do (Suh et al., 1998). Given these cultural differences, a four-factor model (Family, Friends, School, Living Environment) with Korean students, particularly with preadolescent students who have not reached the developmental stage of identity development (Erikson, 1963) was hypothesized.

METHOD

Participants

Korean participants consisted of 398 students (ages 9–12) from two elementary schools, 198 students (ages 13–15) from two middle schools, and 239 students (ages 16–18) from two high schools. All the schools were located in a mid-sized city of South Korea. Students from regular classrooms in grades 4, 5, 7, 8, 10 and 11 participated in the study. Students in grades 6, 9 and 12 were not included in this research because in Korea, students in the last year of each level of school experience extreme stress due to preparing for very competitive exams required to advance to the next level of schools. Therefore, the life satisfaction of students in those grades might not be typical of students in the same school level in other nations.

Data from American students previously collected in elementary (Huebner, 1994), middle (Huebner et al., 1998) and high (Gilman, 1999) schools in South Carolina were used for cross-cultural comparisons. Among American students who were matched with Korean students by grade and age, 350, 224 and 248 students were in elementary, middle and high school, respectively. Korean elementary groups completed 4-point MSLSS scales for cross-cultural comparisons because available American elementary group data were collected using 4-point scales, whereas middle and high school groups used 6-point scales. The average age of Korean

TABLE I

Participants by grade and gender

School	Grade	Korean (N = 835)			American (N = 822)		
		Male	Female	Total	Male	Female	Total
Elementary	4th	100	84	184	107	74	181
	5th	107	107	214	81	88	169
Middle	7th	29	36	65	38	36	74
	8th	61	72	133	70	80	150
High	10th	36	37	73	39	40	79
	11th	84	82	166	86	83	169
Total		417	418	835	421	401	822

students was 12.85 years, with 49.9% males and 50.1% females. The selected American students had an average age of 12.89 years, with 51.2% males and 48.8% females. Means and standard deviations for each domain and total scores of the MSLSS for the Korean and American samples are presented separately in Table I.

Measures

The Multidimensional Students' Life Satisfaction Scale (MSLSS: Huebner, 1994). The MSLSS is a 40-item self-report scale designed to measure children and adolescents' satisfaction with five life domains: Friends, Family, School, Self, and Living Environment. Two different types of response formats were used in this study. Students of middle and high school level were asked to select one of six options (strongly disagree, moderately disagree, mildly disagree, mildly agree, moderately agree, strongly agree) for each question. For elementary school students, a four-option response format (never, sometimes, often, almost always) was used. This procedure was necessary in order to compare scores of Korean elementary students to those of the corresponding American students who used a four-option response format.

The MSLSS, originally written in English, was translated into Korean for Korean participants by the first author of this study.

The final Korean version of the MSLSS was verified by a bilingual Korean through back translation, which is the recommended procedure for creating semantic equivalence (Benet and Waller, 1995). Before it was used, the Korean version of MSLSS was also reviewed by two Korean teachers at the elementary and middle school levels, who examined the items for developmentally appropriate levels of language and for culturally appropriate expressions.

Procedure

After obtaining approval for the study from the principal of each school, participants were selected from targeted classrooms. Following the conventional ethical guidelines for research in Korea, after obtaining approval for the study from the school administrators and teachers, a letter was sent to all parents informing them of the purpose of the study and the procedures, and giving them the option to deny their children's participation to the study; no parent declined permission. Students were also informed that they could withdraw from the study at any time if they did not want to participate for any reason; no student withdrew. A research assistant and the classroom teachers gave detailed verbal directions for completing the questionnaire to the students and answered students' questions. After completing the instrument, students were debriefed about the purpose of the study.

Data Analyses

Prior to the main analysis, data screening procedures were performed using SAS programs (SAS 6.11; SAS Institute, 1990). For most variables, both univariate skewness and kurtosis were smaller than 1.0, except for the Friend domain among American high school students, where they were 1.5 and 3.2, respectively, and still within acceptable values for normality (Curran et al., 1996; Kline, 1998). Possible multivariate outliers for the data set were then examined through Mahalanobis distance, which measure the multivariate distance between individual scores and the sample means (Kline, 1998). Using the Mahalanobis distance scale with conservative $p < 0.001$ as suggested by Tabachinick and Fidell (1996), no case differed significantly from the others. The squared

Mahalanobis distance of all cases was smaller than 43.8, which was the critical value of $\chi^2(19)$ used in this study.

In order to determine whether the MSLSS measures the same constructs across the two cultural groups, covariance matrices of the MSLSS for each group were compared using a multi-sample confirmatory factor analysis (MCFA).

For this study, item parcels were used instead of individual items as observed variables. Researchers have argued that results based upon individual items are difficult to interpret, even for only moderately lengthy questionnaires (e.g., Floyd and Widaman, 1995; Kishton and Widaman, 1994). Following the method used by Gilman (1999) and Huebner et al. (1998), item parcels were constructed with randomly assigned items with a few conditions. In order to avoid a "bloated specific" effect (Cattell, 1978), items which were the most highly inter correlated were not combined. Also, in order to prevent priming effects, items presented next to each other on the scale were not combined for the same parcel (Gilman, 1999). A total of 18 item parcels were constructed for the MSLSS: Four item parcels for each of the Friends, School, and Living Environment domains, and three item parcels to represent the Family and Self domains (descriptions of each item parcel are presented in Huebner et al., 1998). Due to limitation of space, the correlation matrices for the item parcels are not presented in this paper.

Prior to multigroup invariance analyses, the baseline model was established following the previous confirmatory factor analysis findings from American samples (Gilman, 1999; Huebner et al., 1998). The identified baseline model was the five-factor structure comprising Family, Friends, Self, School, and Living Environment, with the five factors assumed to be intercorrelated. Each item parcel was loaded onto a hypothesized factor.

The hierarchical analytic step which tests models in an orderly sequence is recommended in order to determine factor structure equivalence and to identify the source of any inequivalence across groups by researchers (Byrne, 1994; Keith et al., 1995). In this study, a series of increasingly more restrictive models was specified and tested separately for elementary, middle and high school students. In each model, sets of particular parameters were constrained to be equal across the groups and then that model was compared to a less restrictive model in which the parameters were freed. In this study, the following models were tested in steps:

Model 1: All parameters (i.e., factor loadings, unique and error variances, factor correlations, factor variances) were allowed to vary across groups (i.e., number of factors are same).
Model 2: Only the factor loadings were specified to be equal across groups.
Model 3: Factor loadings and the unique and error variances were specified as invariant across groups. Factor variances and covariances were allowed to vary across groups.
Model 4: Factor loadings, unique and error variances and factor covariances were specified to be equal across groups. Only the factor variances were allowed to vary across groups.
Model 5: All parameters were specified to be equivalent across groups.

In the process of determining factor invariance across groups, following the recommendation of researchers (e.g., Keith et al., 1995), the equivalence of factor loadings across groups was considered the most important condition in this study. However, the equivalence of other aspects of the model across groups was also reviewed to explore other potential source of nonequivalence (Keith et al., 1995; Marsh, 1993). All models were tested with the maximum-likelihood estimation procedure using EQS (Bentler, 1995). Both absolute fit statistics; and incremental fit statistics were utilized to evaluate the model fit (see Hoyle and Painter, 1995; Tanaka, 1993). The absolute fit statistics included the χ^2 test of exact model fit, the root-mean-square error of approximation (RMSEA; Steiger and Lind, 1980). The incremental fit statistics (Hoyle and Painter, 1995) included the Comparative Fit Index (CFI; Bentler, 1990), the Tucker-Lewis Index (TLI; Tucker and Lewis, 1973). A small and insignificant χ^2 suggests a good model fitting because the null hypothesis assumes that the model being tested does fit the data. However, the χ^2 test is not a good indicator of model fit when the sample size is large. With large samples, very minor differences can yield a significant χ^2, indicating the rejection of a good model (Keith and Witta, 1997). Thus, considering the relatively large sample size of this study, the results of the chi-square

TABLE II

Reliability coefficients of the Korean version of the MSLSS scores

	Domain					
	Family	Friends	School	Living environment	Self	Total
Elementary	0.76	0.82	0.81	0.78	0.67	0.90
Middle	0.84	0.87	0.85	0.81	0.80	0.91
High	0.87	0.85	0.87	0.80	0.77	0.92

Elementary: 4-point scale; Middle and High: 6-point scale.

test were not considered to be critical in evaluating model fit for this study. In general, for indices, the CFI and TLI, values greater than 0.95 and for the RMSEA indices, below 0.06 indicate good model fit (Browne and Mels, 1992; Hu and Bentler, 1998; Steiger, 1989). In addition, the χ^2 difference test ($\Delta\chi^2$), which tests the statistically significant change in χ^2 values with difference in degrees of freedom (Δdf) between competing models (Byrne, 1991), was used in evaluations of model fit.

RESULTS

Reliability of Korean Version of the MSLSS

Internal consistency estimates (alpha coefficients) for each domain and total scores of the MSLSS for the Korean samples were computed by school level. Internal consistency reliability indices, alpha coefficients (Cronbach, 1951), for the MSLSS of Korean students are reported in Table II by school level. The results for American samples were comparable and have been reported previously (see Gilman, 1999; Huebner, 1994; Huebner et al., 1998).

For the Korean sample, all alphas except those for the Self domain for the elementary students exceeded the value of 0.70 which is considered adequate for research purposes (Nunnally, 1978; Schmitt, 1996). The alphas for the Total MSLSS scores were 0.90 or higher across all school levels of Korean students. These results are consistent with research findings with American students (Huebner, 1994, 1998; Huebner et al., 1998) and Canadian students (Greenspoon and Saklofske, 1997). However, the alpha for the Self subscale among Korean elementary students was 0.67, slightly below but still close to the acceptable range. According to subsequent analyses, the item "I like to try new things" had the smallest item-total correlation ($r = 0.12$ for elementary, $r = 0.31$ for middle, $r = 0.26$ for high school) among the Self items, indicating that this item may not measuring the same construct measured by the other items in the Self subscale. Across all levels of Korean students, the Self subscale demonstrated higher reliability after removing this item ($\alpha = 0.71$: elementary, 0.82: middle, 0.79: high school).

Thus, these results demonstrated adequate internal consistency of the Korean version of the MSLSS Total and subscale scores, except for the slightly lower level of reliability for the Self domain. This finding suggested cautious interpretation of the Self domain score for Korean elementary students.

Factor Structure Equivalence of MSLSS Across Cultural Groups

Following the steps described previously, the results of the series of tests for the comparison of factor models for Korean and American students are summarized in Table III by school level.

For the elementary school level, Model 2, which specified that all factor loadings were equal across the Korean and American students, produced overall good fit statistics, although the fit was slightly decreased when compared to that of Model 1, which freed all parameters. However, the chi-square difference test was statistically significant ($\Delta\chi^2_{(13)} = 26.189, p < 0.05$). These results indicated that there may be problems in constraining equality of factor loadings of certain item parcels across groups. Further analysis of univariate Lagrange Multiplier (LM) χ^2 test results indicated that the factor loading of one item parcel (FRI 2) on the Friend factor was not equal across groups ($p < 0.05$). The standardized factor loadings for Model 2 are presented in Table IV by groups and school level.

The result indicated a slightly higher factor loading for the Korean sample (0.82 vs. 0.78). However, freeing this parameter did not improve model fit significantly. When the model gradually added more constraints across groups, such as unique and error variance, and factor covariances and variances, the overall model

TABLE III

Comparisons of the fit of factor models specifying degrees of equivalence across Korean and American students

Model tested	CFI	TLI	RMSEA	$\chi^2(df)$	$\Delta\chi^2(df)$
Elementary school (4-point scale)					
1. All parameters vary	0.969	0.963	0.032	388.768 (250)	
2. Only factor loadings equal	0.967	0.961	0.033	414.957 (263)	26.189 (13)*
3. Factor loadings and unique/ error variances equal	0.954	0.950	0.037	488.602 (281)	73.645 (18)**
4. Factor loadings, unique/error variances and factor covariances equal	0.951	0.949	0.037	512.450 (291)	23.848 (10)**
5. All parameters invariant	0.948	0.947	0.038	530.514 (296)	18.064 (5)**
Middle school (6-point scale)					
1. All parameters vary	0.949	0.937	0.043	440.047 (250)	
2. Only factor loadings equal	0.947	0.938	0.043	461.324 (263)	21.277 (13)
3. Factor loadings and unique/ error variances equal	0.923	0.916	0.049	568.177 (281)	106.853 (18)**
4. Factor loadings, unique/error variances and factor covariances equal	0.921	0.916	0.049	585.649 (291)	17.472 (10)
5. All parameters invariant	0.913	0.910	0.051	617.613 (296)	31.964 (5)**
High school (6-point scale)					
1. All parameters vary	0.955	0.945	0.040	450.995 (250)	
2. Only factor loadings equal	0.950	0.942	0.042	488.560 (263)	37.565 (13)**
3. Factor loadings and unique/ error variances equal	0.914	0.906	0.053	667.542 (281)	78.982 (18)**
4. Factor loadings, unique/error variances and factor covariances equal	0.909	0.905	0.053	698.433 (291)	30.891 (10)**
5. All parameters invariant	0.901	0.897	0.055	742.499 (296)	44.066 (5)**

$^{*}p < 0.05$; $^{**}p < 0.01$.

fit indices slightly decreased compared to less restrictive models, but they still indicated good model fit. Thus, these results indicated factor invariance of MSLSS across cultural groups at the elementary school level.

For the middle school level, the fit indices for Model 2 indicated a fairly good fit. When Model 2 was compared to Model 1,

TABLE IV

Standardized factor loadings for Model 2: Only factor loadings are equal across Korean and American groups

Item parcel	Elementary		Middle		High	
	K	A	K	A	K	A
FAM1	0.838	0.906	0.838	0.912	0.911	0.902
FAM2	0.641	0.660	0.641	0.704	0.745	0.757
FAM3	0.631	0.741	0.631	0.765	0.735	0.788
FRI1	0.556	0.510	0.556	0.622	0.611	0.526
FRI2	0.820	0.776	0.820	0.849	0.865	0.845
FRI3	0.789	0.885	0.789	0.855	0.878	0.839
FRI4	0.734	0.737	0.734	0.760	0.801	0.720
SCH1	0.780	0.820	0.780	0.773	0.851	0.814
SCH2	0.747	0.838	0.747	0.832	0.866	0.880
SCH3	0.778	0.798	0.778	0.752	0.798	0.735
SCH4	0.732	0.734	0.732	0.748	0.752	0.770
LIV1	0.769	0.837	0.769	0.807	0.857	0.823
LIV2	0.673	0.776	0.673	0.750	0.728	0.751
LIV3	0.742	0.807	0.742	0.660	0.759	0.709
LIV4	0.662	0.748	0.662	0.726	0.613	0.660
SELF1	0.736	0.814	0.736	0.832	0.771	0.898
SELF2	0.559	0.677	0.559	0.749	0.641	0.761
SELF3	0.637	0.731	0.637	0.695	0.722	0.772

K = Korean; A = American.
Unstandardized loadings are constrained to be equal across-groups in MCFA.

the χ^2 difference between these models was statistically insignificant ($\Delta\chi^2_{(13)} = 21.277$, $p > 0.05$), indicating noninvariance of factor loadings across groups. There was a significant decrease in model fit from Model 2 to Model 3, but both models remained in the range of acceptable model fit. These results indicated that the unique and error variances of measurement may not be equivalent across groups. In additional model testing, when the equal factor covariance constraints were introduced on Model 2, the test results showed that the pattern of factor correlations was equivalent across groups ($\Delta\chi^2_{(10)} = 16.602$, $p > 0.05$).

For the high school level, the fit statistics for Model 2 showed a well-fitting model. However, the difference in χ^2 between Model 1 and 2 was statistically significant ($\Delta\chi^2_{(13)} = 37.565$, $p < 0.01$), indicating possible nonequivalence of some factor loadings across groups. Further investigation with univariate LM χ^2 reported that factor loadings of four item parcels (e.g., SCH2, LIV2, LIV3, LIV4) were statistically different between groups ($p < 0.05$). However, the differences appeared to be minor so that freeing these parameters did not change the model fit significantly. When Model 3 was tested, the fit indices showed a substantial decrease compared to Model 2, although the fit was still acceptable. It indicated that the unique and error variances of item parcels were significantly different across groups.

In summary, MCFA results demonstrated that the factor structure of the MSLSS was very similar across Korean and American students at all school levels (elementary, middle and high school). Although, the factor loadings of some item parcels showed differences across cultures at elementary and high school levels, the differences were very marginal. This indicated that the MSLSS measures the same five constructs (i.e., Family, School, Friends, Living Environment, Self) across Korean and American groups.

DISCUSSION

There has been an evident need for cross-cultural research to investigate contextual influences on the psychological processes underlying subjective well-being among children and adolescents. However, the common strategy of comparing mean scores of translated measures across cultural groups is potentially misleading if the constructs being measured differ across groups. Therefore, for valid research on cultural differences in the life satisfaction of students, the demonstration of measurement equivalence across cultures is a prerequisite (Byrne, 1996; Little, 1997). In the present study, the cultural comparability of the psychometric properties of MSLSS was investigated with Korean and American students in elementary, middle, and high schools.

The results of this study provide substantial evidence for the reliability of the Korean version of the MSLSS across all three school levels. Except the Self domain for elementary students, the internal consistency coefficients for the MSLSS total and domain scores were found to be acceptable for research purposes across all levels of Korean students (Schmitt, 1996). These results were consistent with findings from previous research with Canadian students (Greenspoon and Saklofske, 1997), Spanish students (Casas et al., 2001) and American students (Huebner, 1994, 1998). However, the Self domain in Korean elementary school students did not reach an acceptable reliability, although it was quite close. Furthermore, the Self domain showed the lowest reliability estimates within each school level. Thus, it is suggested that caution be taken when interpreting Self domain scores for Korean students, particularly elementary students. Subsequent analyses revealed that removing one item "I like to try new things" from the Self domain increased the alpha coefficient across all school levels. For future research, it is suggested that this item be excluded or modified in order to have a more reliable MSLSS for use with Korean students.

Also, the internal consistency estimates for Korean students were slightly higher at the middle and high school levels than at the elementary school level. These findings may be due to the differences of response scales (4-point for elementary vs. 6-point for middle and high) of the MSLSS. They may also mean that secondary school students have a more well-developed ability to evaluate themselves consistently in specific life domains due to advanced cognitive maturity, which is crucial for valid self-reports. Therefore, future research should investigate possible developmental influences on life satisfaction judgments.

The current study demonstrated that the overall factor structure of the MSLSS was equivalent across Korean and American students at all school levels. This finding suggests that the MSLSS measures the same five constructs (Family, School, Friends, Living Environment, Self) in both Korean and American groups. Thus, the results of cross-cultural comparisons of MSLSS scores can be interpreted in meaningful ways.

This result was not anticipated from the hypothesis which predicted a four-factor structure (Family, School, Friends, Living Environment) for Korean students. This hypothesis was based on the collectivistic nature of the Korean culture which emphasizes the interdependent self (Suh et al., 1998). The current findings indicated that Korean students were able to differentiate their satisfaction in the five life domains in the same way American students did. These findings are similar to research on Chinese students' self-concepts, which demonstrated that Chinese children differentiated their competence in different areas as did their American counterparts (Stigler et al., 1985).

These results suggest that although Korean students from collectivistic societies tend to rely more on the group's norms and see themselves in relation to others than do students from individualistic cultures (Markus and Kitayama, 1991; Suh et al., 1998), they are still able to differentiate their experience of an independent self from an interdependent self both before and during adolescence. Other research similarly found that Chinese students distinguish between the two selves (Violato and Kwok, 1995).

Most importantly, the present findings showed that Korean students differentiated five salient life satisfaction domains included in the current MSLSS in the same manner as USA students. Thus, the findings suggest the generalizability of the multidimensional framework underlying the MSLSS to the Korean culture. However, alternative multidimensional models might also be useful to address some research questions. There might be other domains of life satisfaction or aspects of life satisfaction that may better represent one cultural group compared to others. For example, the Self domain of the MSLSS may emphasize aspects which are more important for Americans than Koreans. Individual items comprising the Self domain of the MSLSS may be tapping personal or independent aspects of the self, which are relatively less important in collectivistic cultures such as Korea, where the group related, interdependent and social self seems to be more important (Markus and Kitayama, 1991; Suh et al., 1998). Thus, further cross-cultural research including items tapping the collectivistic self as well as the individualistic self and asking about culturally sensitive life satisfaction domains need to be done in order to understand possible cultural differences in the nature and determinants of students' overall life satisfaction.

Also, attention needs to be paid to the handful of item parcels that had different factor loadings across the two cultures, although the differences were very small. Cautious interpretation of the Friends domain score for the elementary school sample and the School and Living Environment scores for high school sample are recommended when these scores are compared across cultures. Also, further study is needed to tease out the specific source of these differences, as data artifacts or genuine cultural differences.

In conclusion, the current study provides cross-cultural support for the MSLSS as a reliable and valid measure of life satisfaction in elementary through high school students in Korea and US. More cross-cultural investigations on the factor structure equivalency of the MSLSS need to be carried out with various samples from different cultural backgrounds in order to further validate current research findings. Culturally equivalent measurement is a prerequisite for further investigation into cultural influences on the nature of life satisfaction among children and adolescents.

REFERENCES

Basic Behavioral Science Task Force of the National Advisory Mental Health Council: 1996, 'Basic behavioral science research for mental health: sociocultural and environmental processes', American Psychologist 51, pp. 722–731.

Benet, V. and N.G. Waller: 1995, 'The Big Seven factor model of personality description: Evidence for its cross-cultural generality in a Spanish sample', Journal of Personality and Social Psychology 69, pp. 701–718.

Bentler, P.M.: 1990, 'Comparative fit indexes in structural models', Psychological Bulletin 107, pp. 238–246.

Bentler, P.M.: 1995, EQS: Structural Equations Program Manual (Multivariate Software, Encico, CA).

Bond, M.H. and Task-sking: 1983, 'College students' spontaneous self-concept', Journal of Cross-Cultural Psychology 14, pp. 153–171.

Byrne, B.M.: 1991, 'The Maslach inventory; validating factorial structure and invariance across intermediate, secondary, and university educators', Multivariate Behavioral Research 26, pp. 583–605.

Byrne, B.M.: 1994, 'Burnout: Testing for the validity, replication, and invariance of causal structure across elementary, intermediate, and secondary teachers', American Educational Research Journal 31, pp. 645–673.

Byrne, B.M.: 1996, Measuring Self-concept across the Life Span: Issues and Instrumentation (American Psychological Association, Washington, DC).

Casas, F., C. Alsinet, M. Rosich, E.S. Huebner and J.E. Laughlin: 2001, 'Cross-cultural investigation of the Multidimensional Students' Life Satisfaction Scale with Spanish adolescents', in F. Casas and C. Saurina (eds.), Proceedings of the Third Conference of the International Society for Quality of Life Studies (University of Girona Press, Girona, Spain), pp. 359–366.

Cronbach, L.J.: 1951, 'Coefficient alpha and the internal structure of tests', Psychometrika 16, pp. 297–334.

Curran, P.J., S.G. West and J.F. Finch: 1996, 'The robustness of test statistics to nonnormality and specification error in confirmatory factor analysis', Psychological Methods 1, pp. 16–29.

Diener, E. and M. Diener: 1995, 'Cross-cultural correlates of life satisfaction and self-esteem', Journal of Personality and Social Psychology 68, pp. 653–663.

Floyd, F.J. and K.F. Widaman:1995, 'Factor analysis in the development and refinement of clinical assessment instruments', Psychological Assessment 7, pp. 286–299.

Furr, R.M. and D.C. Funder: 1998, 'A multimodal analysis of personal negativity', Journal of Personality and Social Psychology 74, pp. 1580–1591.

Gilman, R.C.: 1999, Validation of the multidimensional students' life satisfaction scale with adolescents, unpublished doctoral dissertation, University of South Carolina, Columbia.

Gilman, R., E.S. Huebner and J.E. Laughlin: 2000, 'A first study of the Multidimensional Students' Life Satisfaction Scale with high school students', Social Indicators Research 52, pp. 135–160.

Greenspoon, P.J. and D.H. Saklofske: 1997, 'Validity and reliability of the Multidimensional Students' Life Satisfaction Scale with Canadian children', Journal of Psychoeducational Assessment 15, pp. 138–155.

Hoyle, R.H. and A.T. Painter: 1995, 'Writing about structural equation models', in R.H. Hoyle (ed.), Structural Equation Modeling; Concepts, Issues, and Applications (Sage, Thousand Oaks, CA).

Hu, L. and P.M. Bentler: 1998, 'Fit indices in covariance structure modeling: Sensitivity to underparameterized model misspecification', Psychological Methods 3, pp. 424–453.

Huebner, E.S.: 1994, 'Preliminary development and validation of a multidimensional life satisfaction scale for children', Psychological Assessment 6, pp. 149–158.

Huebner, E.S.: 1998, 'Cross-racial application of a children's multidimensional life satisfaction scale', School Psychology International 19, pp. 179–188.

Huebner, E.S., J.E. Laughlin, C. Ash and R. Gilman: 1998, 'Development of a new measure of children's psychological well-being: Further validation of the multidimensional Students' Life Satisfaction Scale', Journal of Psychoeducational Assessment 16, pp. 118–134.

Keith, T.Z., M.H. Fugate, M. DeGraff, C.M. Diamond, E.A. Shadrach and M.L. Setvens: 1995, 'Using multi-sample confirmatory factor analysis to test for construct bias: An example using the K-ABC', Journal of Psychoeducational Assessment 13, pp. 347–364.

Keith, T.Z. and E.L. Witta: 1997, 'Hierarchical and cross-age confirmatory factor analysis of the WISC-III: What does it measure?', School Psychology Quarterly 12, pp. 89–107.

Kishton, J.M. and K.F. Widaman: 1994, 'Unidimensional versus domain representative parceling of questionnaire items: An empirical example', Educational and Psychological Meeasurement 54, pp. 757–765.

Kline, R.B.: 1998, Principles and Practice of Structural Equation Modeling (The Guilford Press, New York).

Lewinsohn, P., J. Redner and J. Seeley: 1991, 'The relationship between life satisfaction and psychosocial variables: New perspectives', in F. Strack, M. Argyle and N. Schwarz (eds.), Subjective Well-being: An Interdisplinary Perspective (Pergamon Press, Oxford), pp. 141–172.

Little, T.D.: 1997, 'Mean and Covariance Structures (MACS) analyses of cross-cultural data: Practical and Theoretical issues', Multivariate Behavioral Research 32, pp. 53–76.

Little, T.D.:2000, 'On the comparability of constructs in cross-cultural research: A critique of Cheung and Rensvold', Journal of Cross-cultural psychology 31, pp. 213–219.

Man, P.: 1991, 'The influence of peers and parents on youth life satisfaction in Hong Kong', Social Indicators Research 24, pp. 347–365.

Markus, H.R. and S. Kitayama: 1991, 'Cultural variation in the self-concept', in J. Strauss and G.R. Goethals (eds.), The Self: Interdisciplinary Approaches (Springer-Verlag, New York), pp. 18–48.

Markus, H.R. and S. Kitayama: 1994, 'A collective fear of the collectives: Implications for selves and theories of selves', Personality and Social Psychology Bulletin 20, pp. 568–579.

Meredith, W.: 1993, 'Measurement invariance, factor analysis and factorial invariance', Psychometrika 58, pp. 525–543.

Nunally, J.C.: 1978, Psychometric Theory, 2nd ed. (McGraw-Hill, New York).

Riordan, C.M. and R.J. Vandenberg: 1994, 'A central question in cross-cultural research: Do employees of different cultures interpret work-related measures in a equivalent manner?', Journal of Management 20, pp. 643–671.

SAS Institute, Inc.: 1990, The CALIS Procedure: Analysis of Covariance Structures (SAS Institute, Cary, NC).

Schmitt, N.: 1996, 'Uses and abuses of coefficient alpha', Psychological Assessment 8, pp. 350–353.

Strack, F., M. Argyle and N. Schwarz: 1991, Subjective Well-being: An Interdisplinary Perspective (Pergamon Press, Oxford).

Steiger, J.H.: 1989, EZPATH. A Supplementary Module for SYSTAT and SYSGRAPH (SYSTAT, Evanstan, IL).

Steiger, J.H. and J.C. Lind: 1980, 'Statistically based tests for the number of factors', paper presented at the annual meeting of the Psychometric Society, Iowa City, IA.

Stigler, J.W., S. Smith and L. Mao: 1985, 'The self-perception of competence by Chinese children', Child Development 56, pp. 1259–1270.

Suh, E., E. Diener, S. Oishi and H.C. Triandis: 1998, 'The shifting basis of life satisfaction judgments across cultures: Emotions versus norms', Journal of Personality and Social Psychology 74, pp. 482–493.

Tabachinick, B.G. and L.S. Fidell: 1996, Using Multivariate Statistics, 3rd ed. (Haper Collins, New York).
Tanaka, J.S.: 1993, 'Multifaceted conceptions of fit in structural equation models', in K.A. Bollen and J.S. Long (eds.), Testing Structural Equation Models (Sage, Newbury Park, CA), pp. 10–39.
Tucker, L.R. and C. Lewis: 1973, 'A reliability coefficient for maximum likelihood factor analysis', Psychometrika 38, pp. 1–10.
Veenhoven, R.: 1996, 'Developments in satisfaction research', Social Indicators Research 37, pp. 1–46.
Violato, C. and D. Kwok: 1995, 'A cross-cultural validation of a four-factor model of adolescent concerns: A confirmatory factor analysis based on a sample of Hong Kong Chinese adolescents', Journal of Adolescence 18, pp. 607–617.

Department of Psychology
University of Rhode Island
Kingston, RI 02881
USA
E-mail: npark@uri.edu

Nansook Park

University of South Carolina
Columbia, SC
USA

E. Scott Huebner
James E. Laughlin
Robert F. Valois

University of Kentucky
Lexington, KY
USA

Rich Gilman

ROBERT F. VALOIS, KEITH J. ZULLIG, E. SCOTT HUEBNER and J. WANZER DRANE

LIFE SATISFACTION AND SUICIDE AMONG HIGH SCHOOL ADOLESCENTS

ABSTRACT. Relationships between perceived life satisfaction, poor mental health, suicide ideation and suicide behaviors were examined in a statewide sample of 13 to 18 year old public high school students (n = 4,758) using the self-report CDC Youth Risk Behavior Survey (YRBS). Adjusted logistic regression analyses and multivariate models constructed separately (via SUDAAN), revealed that poor mental health (past 30 days), poor mental/physical health (past 30 days) serious suicide consideration (past 12 months), planning for suicide (past 12 months), attempted suicide (past 12 months) and suicide attempt requiring medical care (past 12 months) were significantly related to reduced life satisfaction. Also, differences across gender and race were demonstrated. Measures of life satisfaction as a component of comprehensive assessments of adolescent mental health, suicide ideation and suicide behavior in fieldwork, research, and program-evaluation efforts should be considered.

KEY WORDS: adolescents, mental health, perceived life satisfaction, quality of life, suicide

INTRODUCTION

Suicide currently ranks as the third leading cause of death among 15- to 24-year-olds in the USA, exceeded only by injuries and homicides (Hoyert, Kochannek and Murphy, 1999). In 1997, the year with the most current mortality statistics, the suicide rate among this age group was 11.4 per 1000,000. the suicide rate for adolescents has more than tripled since the 1950's while the rates for the overall population has remained virtually unchanged. A typical USA high school classroom includes one male and two females who attempted suicide in the past year (King, 1997). The US Department of Health and Human Services (1991) designated the reduction of adolescent suicides to less than 8.2 per 100,000 and the reduction of injuries associated with suicide attempts by 15% as goals to be

Social Indicators Research **66:** 81–105, 2004.

achieved by the year 2000. The 1999 Surgeon General's Call to Action to Prevent Suicide (USPHS, 1991) reiterated the urgency to treat suicide as a serious public health problem. Thus, suicide prevention among adolescents remains a major health promotion issue in the USA.

According to some theorists (Deiner, 2000; Raphael, 1996) the cornerstone of health promotion is the enhancement of quality of life (QOL). Research bridging health-related behavior and QOL has been scarce, although some particularly noteworthy efforts have been published (Renwick, Brown and Nagler, 1996). This article considers whether one crucial aspect of QOL, that is, "life satisfaction", is associated with suicide ideation and suicide behavior among adolescents. Specifically, it provides an empirical test of the hypothesis that life-satisfaction reports are associated with adolescent mental health, suicide ideation and suicidal behavior. The findings subsequently contribute to consideration of the implications of QOL research for health promotion theory, practice, and research involving adolescents.

Quality-of-life research has been conceptualized from two perspectives: objective and subjective. The objective perspective focuses on external conditions that contribute to quality of life, such as income levels, housing quality, friendship networks, and access to health services. In contrast, subjective QOL refers to individuals' internal judgments of their quality of life. Subjective QOL includes, but is not limited to a person's life satisfaction judgments, with respect to overall lives and/or specific life domains (e.g., satisfaction with friends, family, school experiences) (Deiner et al., 1999; Huebner, 1997). In the development of their QOL model, Day and Jankey (1996) concluded, that although objective life circumstances are important in individuals' determination of the quality of their lives, their subjective interpretations and evaluations of their experiences are most crucial.

Life satisfaction has been defined as a cognitive evaluation of the quality of a person's overall life or with specific aspects of life, such as family, friends, and community (Pavot et al., 1991). Accordingly, individuals' overall life satisfaction reports are based upon personal comparisons between self-determined criteria and perceived life circumstances. Similarly, life satisfaction refers to "a person's subjective evaluation of the degree to which his or her most important needs, goals, and wishes have been fulfilled" (Frisch, 1998: p. 24). Overall life satisfaction is expected to influence the probability of subsequent emotional and behavioral responses in relation to particular life events (Deiner, 1994; Lazarus, 1991). Thus, although demonstrating a degree of short-term and long-term stability, (Gilman and Huebner, 1997; Huebner, Funk and Gilman, 2000), changes in global life-satisfaction may elicit changes in adolescents coping strategics. For example, some individuals might respond to declines in life satisfaction and associated emotions by engaging in various risk-taking behaviors related to health (e.g., suicide ideation and suicide attempts).

Historically, life-satisfaction research has been mostly limited to studies of adults (Veenhoven, 1988). During the past decade, however, increasing attention has been paid to the determinants, correlates, and consequences of individual differences in life satisfaction among children and adolescents (Huebner, 1997). Global life-satisfaction reports of adolescents have been related to a variety of variables, including environmental variables (Ash and Huebner, 2001; McCullough et al., 2000), demographic variables, such as socioeconomic status (SES) (Dew and Huebner, 1994; Huebner et al., 2000), and personality and temperament variables (Fogle, Huebner and Laughlin, in press; Huebner, 1991; Huebner and Alderman, 1994). Life-satisfaction measures have been found to be related, but separate from traditional measures of mental health (Deiner et al., 1999; Huebner et al., 2000). Efforts to measure life satisfaction have been consistent with the positive mental-health orientation that defines psychological well-being as more than the absence of psychopathological symptoms (Frisch, 2000; Seligman and Csikszentmihalyi, 2000). That is, an individual can be dissatisfied with life as a result of experiencing undesirable circumstances, yet not display symptoms of psychopathology. Similarly, an individual may be relatively satisfied with her or his life, but concurrently experience symptoms. Nevertheless, perceived life satisfaction for adolescents has been found to be associated with various health risk behaviors, including alcohol and other drug use (Clark and Kirisci, 1996; Newcomb et al., 1986; Zullig et al., 2000), violent and aggressive behaviors (Valois et al., 2001), dating violence (Coker et al., 2000) and sexual risk-taking behaviors (Valois et al., 2002).

A review of literature yielded little research devoted to investigating the relationship between life satisfaction and suicide ideation and/or suicide behaviors and life satisfaction among adults and/or youth. Two studies of adults and one with adolescents suggest links between suicide and life satisfaction. From a nationwide sample of adults aged 18–24 in Finland, using a 20-year follow up technique, Koivumaa-Honkanen et al. (2001), found that life dissatisfaction had a long-term effect on the risk of suicide, however, this effect appeared to be partly mediated through poor health behavior. This study also suggested that life satisfaction measures provided an effective composite health indicator. In another study with adults, Lester (1988) examined the associations between suicide rates and life satisfaction in college students from 18 nations. Of the ten correlations between suicide and life satisfaction domains (e.g., satisfaction with friends, family, self, life), only one correlation was significant (i.e., female suicide rate and satisfaction with family). It should be noted that both studies with adults included measures of life satisfaction of unknown validity.

In a path analytic study of adolescents, Thatcher et al. (2002) found that life satisfaction variables mediated the relationships between suicide and some risk behaviors (e.g., drug use) for males. However, the data analytic procedure for this study was limited in that this CDC YRBS data set required the use of SUDAAN (Shah et al., 1996) to most appropriately model the data, vis-a-vis the complex sampling technique and weighted data. In turn, significant amounts of variance remained unaccounted for in the analyses; estimates of association would have likely been more reliable had the appropriate statistical analysis techniques been applied to these data.

Therefore, much work needs to be done to reliably determine the magnitude and meaning of the association between perceived life satisfaction to suicide ideation or suicide behavior among adolescents. Alcohol, tobacco and other drug use, violent behavior and sexual risk-taking have been found to be associated with reduced life satisfaction. It is likely that suicide ideation and suicidal behaviors will prove to be associated with life satisfaction in varying degrees. Therefore, the purpose of this study was to investigate the relationship between life satisfaction and self-reported suicide ideation and suicide behaviors among public high school adolescents in South Carolina public high schools. Also, the association between adolescent life satisfaction reports and reports of mental health and mental/physical health were investigated. Specifically the null hypotheses for this study were that there would be no statistically significant differences in reports of poor mental health (past 30 days), suicide ideation and suicidal behaviors of adolescents who are satisfied with their life and those who are not satisfied with their life.

Our study extended beyond previous research by: (1) focusing on adolescents in USA; (2) using a well-validated measure of life satisfaction; and (3) applying the proper statistical techniques of a large, random, stratified cross-sectional sample with weighted data.

METHODS

Participants

The 1997 South Carolina Youth Risk Behavior Survey (SCYRBS) used a sampling procedure designed to obtain a representative sample (with the exception of special education schools) of all public high school students 13 to 18 years old, in grades 9 through 12, from March until June 1997. The survey questionnaire was previously determined to have adequate reliability (Brenner et al., 1995). The CDC Youth Risk Behavior Surveillance System (YRBSS) focuses on 6 major areas of adolescent behaviors: those that lead to intentional and unintentional injuries; tobacco, alcohol and other drug use; sexual behaviors, dietary behaviors; and physical inactivity (Kolbe, 1990). Schools were randomly selected using a systematic basis for each enrollment-size category, by PCSAMPLE, a computerized sampling program which narrowed the 215 schools to 87 schools in 53 districts, statewide. The 215 schools were stratified by enrollment size into 3 enrollment categories: schools with 74 to 874 students were classified as small; schools with enrollments from 875 to 1,278 were classified as medium; and schools of more than 1,278 were classified as large. Our data are reported on 63 of the 87 eligible schools (72% response rate). Classes that met during second period were eligible for classroom-level sampling selection to maximize student eligibility. Using random starts, classes were selected with a systematic, equal probability sampling. When the number of students selected by PCSAMPLE was substantially less than expected, class samples were increased by the same systematic sampling of additional classes. The desired number of participants (*n* = 125) was met by most schools with the majority of schools sampling between 115 and 145 students. The survey questionnaire was anonymous in that no personal identification was recorded. School and class codes were used for CDC reporting purposes. Parent-notification forms were distributed at least five days in advance of survey administration; those parents who do not want their children to participate were required to return the form. Survey administrations were conducted by trained data collectors, emphasizing anonymity, privacy, and confidentiality. This research was approved by the referent university's review board for the rights of human subjects in research.

Description of Participants

The total number of subjects who participated in the 1997 South Carolina YRBS was 5544 (Table I). However, only 4758 valid observations were available owing to (a) nonresponse by subjects to the variables of interest, (b) responses that could not be read, (c) out-of-range responses, and (d) exclusion of subjects reporting their race as "Other" than black or white (*n* = 388, 7.77%). Failure to answer any risk-variable-of-interest question also resulted in deletion (*n* = 125, 2.48%). Two thousand five hundred and thirty (53.2%) survey participants were female whereas 2228 (46.8%) were male. The study consisted of 2210 (46.4%) black students and 2548 (53.6%) white students. White females accounted for the largest population (27.1%) followed by black females (26.1%) white males (26.4% each) and black males (20.4%).

Instrumentation

The Brief Multidimensional Students' Life Satisfaction Scale (BMSLSS: Seligson et al., 2003) was included in the 1997 South Carolina YRBS. The BMSLSS was based on the 40-item Multidimensional Students Life Satisfaction Scale (Gilman et al.,

TABLE I

Demographic characteristics of the sample

Variable	n	Weighted percentage
Females	2530	53.2%
Males	2228	46.8%
Whites	2548	53.6%
Blacks	2210	46.4%
White females	1290	27.1%
Black females	1240	26.1%
White males	1258	26.4%
Black males	970	20.4%
Grade 9	1624	34.1%
Grade 10	1183	24.9%
Grade 11	1052	22.1%
Grade 12	896	18.8%*

This study analyzed Black and White respondents only $n = 4758$.
Subjects other than Black or White were eliminated.
*Grade was missing for 3 subjects. N = 4755.

2000; Huebner et al., 1998; Huebner, 1994) which measures satisfaction with family, friends, school, self, living environment, and overall life. The BMSLSS has been validated with adolescents through a variety of convergent and discriminant validity procedures (Seligson et al., 2003). The BMSLSS included five items, one for each of the five specific life domains tapped by the MSLSS (e.g., family, friends). One additional item was added to tap satisfaction with life as a whole. The six items in this version of the scale were, "I would describe my satisfaction with my family life as"; "I would describe my satisfaction with my friendships as"; "I would describe my satisfaction with my school experience as"; "I would describe my satisfaction with myself as"; "I would describe my satisfaction with where I live as"; and a global question "I would describe my satisfaction with my overall life as". Seven response options from the widely used Terrible-Delighted Scale (Andrews and Withey, 1976) were used for each of these questions: (a) terrible, (b) unhappy, (c) mostly dissatisfied, (d) mixed (equally satisfied and dissatisfied), (e) mostly satisfied, (f) pleased, and (g) delighted.

The four items from the South Carolina Youth Risk Behavior Survey examined in this study were: (1) During the past 12 months, did you ever seriously consider attempting suicide (yes or no); (2) During the past 12 months, did you make a plan about how you would attempt suicide (yes or no); (3) During the past 12 months, how many times did you actually attempt suicide (0, 1, 2, or 3, 4 or 5, 6 or more times); and (4) If you attempted suicide during the past 12 months, did any attempt result in an injury, poisoning, or overdose that had to be treated by a doctor or nurse (I did not attempt suicide during the past 12 months, yes, no).

Items measuring mental health and mental/physical health are from the four item Health Related Quality of Life Scale (HRQOLS) developed for telephone interviews by Hennessy et al. (1994), validated with adults by Newschaffer (1998) and Morarity and Zack (1999) and modified and validated for paper and pencil survey of adolescents by Zullig et al. (2002). The alpha coefficient for the adolescent study by Zullig et al. (2002) was 0.70. The four HRQOL scale items were: (1) In general, how would you describe your health (excellent, very good, good, fair, poor); (2) Now thinking about your physical health [which includes physical illness and injury], for how many days during the past 30 days was your physical health not good (0, 1–2, 3–5, 6–9, 10–19, 20–29, all 30 days); (3) Now thinking about your mental health [which includes stress, depression and problems with emotions], for how many days during the past 30 days was your mental health not good (0, 1–2, 3–5, 6–9, 10–19, 20–29, all 30 days); and (4) During the past 30 days, on how many days did your poor physical or mental health keep you from doing your usual activities such as school, recreation, or work (0, 1–2, 3–5, 6–9, 10–19, 20–29, all 30 days). Our study utilized two items, mental health days not good (past 30 days) and poor mental/physical health (past 30 days).

Data Analysis

All six discrete variables from the life-satisfaction scale were pooled to form a pseudo-continuous independent variable ranging in score from 6 (1×6) to 42 (7×6). The satisfaction score was expressed as mean satisfaction score (MSS) with lower scores indicative of reduced satisfaction with life. Logistic regression analyses were conducted separately for the four race-gender groups, white females (WF), black females (BF), white males (WM), and black males (BM).

Logistic regression was conducted using SAS-callable Survey Data Analysis (SUDAAN) (Shaw, Barnwell and Beiler, 1996) for weighted data at $\alpha = 0.05$ for this analysis. In addition, SUDAAN takes into account the stratification of schools, clustering within schools and classes nested within schools. The pooled independent variable was collapsed/categorized into the three levels: dissatisfied, midrange, and satisfied adolescents. A numeric collapse of the MSS determined subject classification. MSS scores ranging from 6 to 27 were categorized as dissatisfied; MSS scores ranging from 28 to 34 composed the midrange group; and MSS scores of 35 or greater defined the satisfied group. Odds ratios (OR) and confidence intervals (CI) were calculated to determine which suicide behaviors were associated with reduced life satisfaction for each race-gender group for both the midrange and dissatisfied levels. Students at the satisfied level served as the referent group. Variables that did not meet the 0.05 significance level were not retained in the model. All students who did not answer at least one independent variable question were excluded from the analysis, by the numerical procedures.

The dependent variables explored in this study were: poor mental health days (past 30 days; poor mental or physical health days (past 30 days); serious suicide consideration (past 12 months); planning for suicide (past 12 months); attempted suicide (past 12 months); and suicide attempt requiring medical care (past 12 months) (Table I). Adolescents were categorized as having reported the behavior or not, with the referent group designated as those who did not report involvement in any of the mental health and suicide behaviors. SUDAAN (Shah et al., 1996) automatically deletes any incomplete record. Frequencies and percents for the selected mental health/suicide behaviors are presented in Table II, by race and gender.

TABLE II

Poor mental/physical health, suicide ideation and suicide behavior variables by race/gender group: weighted frequency (*n*) and percent (%)

Risk variable	White females (1341)		Black females (1309)		White males (1309)		Black males (1073)	
	n	(%)	*n*	(%)	*n*	(%)	*n*	(%)
Mental health days not good (past 30 days)								
No days	296	(22.3)	467	(35.7)	552	(47.2)	583	(54.3)
At least 1 day	1043	(20.7)	842	(64.3)	757	(58.7)	490	(45.7)
Mental or physical health days not good (past 30 days)								
No days	644	(48.0)	750	(57.3)	868	(66.3)	701	(65.3)
At least 1 day	697	(52.0)	560	(42.7)	441	(33.7)	372	(34.7)
Seriously considered a plan to Commit suicide (past 12 months)								
No	924	(68.9)	1039	(79.4)	1066	(81.4)	941	(87.7)
Yes	417	(30.1)	270	(20.6)	243	(18.6)	132	(12.3)
Made a plan to attempt suicide (past 12 months)								
No	1053	(78.5)	1113	(85.0)	1112	(85.7)	975	(90.9)
Yes	288	(21.5)	196	(15.0)	187	(14.3)	98	(9.1)
Attempted suicide (past 12 months)								
No	1142	(85.2)	1157	(88.4)	1200	(91.7)	984	(91.7)
At least once	199	(14.8)	152	(11.6)	109	(83.3)	89	(8.3)
Attempted suicide resulting in injury requiring medical care (past 12 months)								
Did not attempt suicide	1142	(85.2)	1157	(88.4)	1200	(91.7)	984	(91.7)
Yes	51	(3.8)	37	(2.6)	31	(2.3)	28	(2.6)
No	148	(11.0)	115	(9.0)	78	(6.0)	61	(5.7)

RESULTS

Perceived Life Satisfaction

A chi-square analysis was performed testing the hypothesis of equal proportions (percentages) across four race-gender groups for levels of life satisfaction (LS) (Table III). An overall chi-square value of

TABLE III

Frequency and weighted percentage perceived life satisfaction level by race and gender

Race and gender	Lower satisfaction	Midrange	Higher satisfaction
White females	351 (26.8%)	542 (42.5%)+	397 (30.7%)
Black females	350 (28.1%)	515 (41.6%)	375 (30.4%)–
White males	324 (25.4%)	486 (38.9%)	448 (35.7%)
Black males	273 (28.2%)	322 (33.2%)–	375 (38.7%)+

$n = 4{,}758$.
– = Significantly low.
+ = Significantly high ($p = 0.10$).
Chi-Square 1df, 0.90 = 2.706 (If cell chi-square > 2.706, declare cell aberrant).
Chi-Square 6df = 32.8, $p = 0.00011$.

32.8 with 6 degrees of freedom with a p-value of 0.000011 was determined. To focus on isolated differences either above or below expectations, cell chi-squares were calculated and tested with an alpha of 0.10 noting observed (O) and expected (E) cases for the cell chi-squares (CCS).

Deviations from expectations were found in white females for midrange LS (O = 557, E = 519, CCS = 2.80, $p = 0.094$), black females high LS (O = 389, E = 430, CCS = 3.91, $p = 0.048$), black males midrange LS (O = 349, E = 415, CCS = 10.5, $p = 0.001$), and black males high LS (O = 395, E = 352, CCS = 513, $p = 0.024$).

Among the 4 race-gender groups, there were no statistical departures from expectations for lower satisfaction. At midrange, white females were over represented (O–E = 38, $p = 0.09$), whereas black males were underrepresented (O–E = –0.66, $p = 0.00001$). Finally, for higher satisfaction, black females were underrepresented (O–E = –41, $p = 0.05$) whereas black males were overrepresented (O–E = 30, $p = 0.02$).

None of the above departures or odds ratios, which could be constructed therefrom, has been adjusted for the risk behaviors located in Table IV.

MIDRANGE LEVEL OF LIFE SATISFACTION, SUICIDE IDEATION AND SUICIDE BEHAVIORS

Logistic regression results here, identified significant "protective" or non-risk associations for the four race-gender groups at the mixed or midrange of life satisfaction. Owing to the lack of risk association between poor mental health, poor mental/physical health; suicide ideation and suicide behavior variables and the midrange level of life satisfaction, these data are neither tabled nor discussed.

LIFE DISSATISFACTION AND SUICIDE IDEATION AND BEHAVIORS

White Females

Significant relationships via logistic regression analysis were established between dissatisfaction with life and poor mental health (past 30 days) (OR = 2.12), poor mental/physical health days (past 30 days) (OR = 2.65), serious suicide consideration (past 12 months) (OR = 6.11), planning for suicide (past 12 months) (OR = 5.36), attempted suicide (past 12 months) (OR = 5.93), and suicide attempt requiring medical care (past 12 months) (OR = 6.65). White adolescent females who reported poor mental health, poor mental/physical health, suicide ideation and suicide behaviors increased the odds of reporting dissatisfaction with their lives by 2.12 to 6.65 times, in comparison to white females who did not report on these mental health/suicide variables.

Black Females

Significant relationships via logistic regression analysis were determined between reported dissatisfaction with life and poor mental health (past 30 days) (OR = 2.14), poor mental/physical health days (past 30 days) (OR = 2.24), serious suicide consideration (past 12 months) (OR = 3.37), planning for suicide (past 12 months) (OR = 3.28), attempted suicide (past 12 months) (OR = 3.07), and suicide attempt requiring medical care (past 12 months) (OR = 3.34). Black adolescent females who reported poor mental health, poor mental/physical health, suicide ideation and suicide behaviors increased the odds of reporting dissatisfaction with their lives by

2.14 to 3.37 times, in comparison to black females who did not report on these mental health/suicide variables.

White Males

Significant relationships via logistic regression analysis were established between dissatisfaction with life and poor mental health (past 30 days) (OR = 2.64), poor mental/physical health days (past 30 days) (OR = 2.55), serious suicide consideration (past 12 months) (OR = 3.85), planning for suicide (past 12 months) (OR = 3.89), attempted suicide (past 12 months) (OR = 7.23), and suicide attempt requiring medical care (past 12 months) (OR = 7.42). White adolescent males who reported poor mental health, poor mental/physical health, suicide ideation and suicide behaviors increased the odds of reporting dissatisfaction with their lives by 2.55 to 7.42 times, in comparison to white males who did not report on these mental health/suicide variables.

Black Males

Significant relationships via logistic regression analysis were determined between reported dissatisfaction with life and poor mental health (past 30 days) (OR = 2.61), poor mental/physical health days (past 30 days) (OR = 2.72), serious suicide consideration (past 12 months) (OR = 2.54), planning for suicide (past 12 months) (OR = 3.27), attempted suicide (past 12 months) (OR = 4.02), suicide attempt requiring medical care (past 12 months) (OR = 1.75). Black adolescent males who reported poor mental health, poor mental/physical health, suicide ideation and suicide behaviors increased the odds of reporting dissatisfaction with their lives by 2.54 to 5.80 times, in comparison to black males who did not report on these mental health/suicide variables.

Discussion

This was a large, cross-sectional study of the association between self-reported life satisfaction and suicide among adolescents. Life satisfaction was measured with an easily administered, six-item scale (Seligson et al., 2003) that assessed satisfaction with family, friends, school, self, living environment and overall life satisfaction (global item).

TABLE IV

Associated poor mental/physical health, suicide ideation and suicide behaviors for race/gender groups at the dissatisfied level of life satisfaction

Risk variable interval	Odds Ratio and 95% Confidence			
	White female	Black female	White male	Black male
Mental health days not good (past 30 days)	2.12**** (1.50–3.00)	2.14** (1.54–2.96)	2.64**** (1.79–3.92)	2.61**** (1.95–3.49)
Mental or physical health days not good (past 30 days)	2.65**** (2.06–3.40)	2.24**** (1.74–2.87)	2.55**** (1.95–3.35)	2.72**** (2.11–3.51)
Seriously considered a plan to commit suicide (past 12 months)	6.11**** (4.31–8.65)	3.37**** (2.67–4.24)	3.85**** (2.67–5.54)	2.54**** (1.73–3.72)
Made a plan to attempt suicide (past 12 months)	5.36**** (3.87–7.42)	3.28**** (2.56–4.20)	3.98**** (2.84–5.59)	3.27**** (1.89–5.67)
Attempted suicide with no need for medical care (past 12 months)	5.66**** (3.62–8.83)	2.81**** (1.96–4.02)	5.79**** (2.74–12.22)	5.80**** (2.87–11.73)
Attempted suicide resulting in injury requiring medical care (past 12 months)	6.65**** (3.62–12.20)	3.34** (1.52–7.34)	7.42**** (3.03–18.17)	1.75 (0.92–3.34)

*$p < 0.05$.
**$p < 0.005$.
***$p < 0.0005$.
****$p < 0.0001$.

Results suggest that a substantial number of public high school students in South Carolina (SC) are reporting dissatisfaction with their lives (Table III). This study also suggests that a substantial number of SC public high school adolescents are experiencing poor mental health days, poor mental/physical health days, suicide ideation and attempted suicide (Table I). Most importantly, this study demonstrated a meaningful linkage between two distinct adolescent health research literatures: the health-risk behavior (intentional injury/suicide) literature and the quality-of-life (life satisfaction) literature. Research efforts bridging the two areas have been scarce; however, this study identified significant relationships between self-reported life satisfaction and poor mental health days, poor mental/physical health days, suicide ideation and suicide behaviors (Table IV). These findings are consistent with the findings of prior research with adults (Koivumma-Honkanen et al., 2001; Lester, 1998). This study thus extends the generalizability of the life dissatisfaction-suicide link to adolescents. Furthermore, this study demonstrated the importance of two contextual factors that influenced the relationship between life satisfaction and suicide behavior. That is, suicide behavior and life satisfaction associations were significantly influenced by student gender and ethnicity.

Adolescent reports of poor mental health days (past 30 days), poor mental/physical health days (past 30 days) serious suicide consideration (past 12 months), planning for suicide (past 12 months), attempted suicide (past 12 months), planning for suicide (past 12 months), attempted suicide (past 12 months), and suicide attempts resulting in injury/requiring medial care appear to associated with life dissatisfaction in this study. Significant relationships were identified between almost all the mental health/suicide variables and dissatisfaction with life at the 0.0001 level of significance in this study. The lone exceptions involved black adolescents. Specifically, the relationship between life satisfaction and attempted suicide resulting in the need for medical care was significant for black females at the 0.005 (vs. 0.0001) level, but not significant for black males.

Several mechanisms might explain the association between adolescent life satisfaction and suicide. One mechanism involves effective coping behavior. Given that life dissatisfaction is related to unfulfilled goals, wishes and needs, coping skills (externalizing behaviors, withdrawal behaviors) among youth (Huebner and Alderman, 1993; Huebner et al., 2000). Difficulties in coping with stress and the challenges of adolescent psychosocial development could mediate the relationship between adolescent life dissatisfaction and suicide. In a general sense, many adolescents are not "life skilled" in five domains: communication, stress management, decision making, problem solving, and goal setting (Valois et al., 1993). Adolescents dissatisfied with life might engage in suicide ideation or suicide behavior as a result of poor communication, decision making and problem solving attempts related to unfulfilled aspirations and needs. Deficiencies in these "life skills" could lead to the inability to cope with various pressures and manage stress, resulting in irrational cognitive judgements, suicide attempts and the subsequent consequences (Garrison et al., 1993). Future research should thus incorporate measures of adolescent coping skills to investigate the potentially complex interrelationships among life satisfaction, coping behavior, and suicide ideation and behavior among adolescents.

Another likely mechanism is social support. Life satisfaction is also strongly associated with social support from family and friends (Dew and Huebner, 1994; Gilman and Huebner, 1997; Huebner, 1991) which in turn is associated with the probability of adolescent depression (Hawkins et al., 1992; Lewinsohn et al., 1991) and suicide ideation and behavior (D'Attilio et al., 1992; Dukes and Lorch, 1989). Sub-clinical levels of life dissatisfaction have been shown to relate to social rejection (Furr and Funder, 1998) among normal college students. Taken together, such findings suggest that levels of social support might mediate the relationship between life dissatisfaction and suicide (and depression as well). Thus, future research is also needed to test the potential mediational role of social support from family and/or friends in the relationship between adolescent life satisfaction and mental health, including depression and suicide behaviors.

IMPLICATIONS

Behavioral health specialists have recently begun to focus greater attention upon the assessment and promotion of youth developmental assets, positive aspects of psychological well-being, and adaption (compass, 1993; Huebner, 1991; Seligman, 1998; Scales, 1999). This focus broadens the matrix of youth assessment beyond those of risk behaviors and psychiatric symptoms (Frisch, 1998; Frisch et al., 1992; Kolbe, 1990; Dryfoos, 1990; Durant et al., 1995), and thus may be more sensitive to subtle, but clinically meaningful changes in adolescent well-being. Subjective life-satisfaction measures can also extend the scope of well-being indicators beyond the objective indicators often used exclusively in federally sponsored large-scale surveys of American children's well-being. For example, one recent federal survey of children entitled *America's Children: Key National Indicators of Well-Being* (Federal Interagency Forum on Child and Family Statistics (1997), was composed entirely of objective indicators such as teenage pregnancies, drug and alcohol usage, and family income. The many potential uses of measures of adolescents' perceptions of their quality of life, such as general and domain-specific life satisfaction measures, have been delineated in a number of sources (Frisch, 1998; Dew and Huebner, 1994; Raphael et al., 1996), including uses in social and health policy formulation, needs assessment, and program evaluation. Thus, human services personnel and researchers working with youth could benefit from including measures of life satisfaction as a component of comprehensive assessments involving correlates of health promoting behaviors in research and evaluation efforts.

Study limitations should be noted here. These limitations include the use of a cross-sectional study where no temporal sequence of reduced life satisfaction as a precursor of suicide behavior can be determined; the use of a geographical sample that may represent youth in this southern USA state, but is not nationally representative; and the elimination of participants with missing data on the variables of interest as required by the SUDAAN (Shah et al., 1996) logistic regression program. Such elimination can introduce biases; however, they are not threatening. The bias is equal to the difference between an estimate using the responders minus the estimate from those not responding times the prevalence of nonresponders (Cochran, 1963).

The study strengths include the large sample size (n = 5,032) the random sampling technique, the stratification of schools by size, good school and class response rates (72% and 88% respectively), reliability and validity of the BMSLSS; the number and types of mental health and suicide variables used; and the analysis of results by race and gender. In addition, the dichotomized variables and associations established between selected mental health and suicide behaviors and life satisfaction could be even stronger and more conservative (i.e., an underestimation of the magnitude of risk and more toward the null hypothesis of no association) than reported.

These results also suggest that comprehensive suicide prevention programs for adolescents are needed. Public schools offer an efficient setting to deliver such services. Such programs should be triangulated among primary, secondary and tertiary prevention program components (King, 2001). Primary prevention should include: Developing a district-wide school policy concerning student suicide; educating school professionals about suicide warning signs and risk factors; encouraging collaboration among a school-based health promotion team (Valois and Hoyle, 2000); including suicide prevention education in the teaching curriculum; developing a peer assistance program; implement activities aimed at increasing school connectedness; fostering supportive school-family and school-community partnerships; and establishing a school crisis intervention team. Secondary prevention (intervention) should include effort to: Ensure student safety; assess the students' suicidal risk; determine mental health services needed; ensure students receive appropriate care; and debrief school staff. Tertiary prevention (postvention) refers to school activities occurring after a student has threatened, attempted or completed suicide. When suicide occurs, it is a traumatic event for many survivors (Leenaars and Wenckstern, 1990). Suicide clusters are well established among adolescents, therefore the school response to an actual suicide is crucial (Capuzzi, 1988). The goal of postvention is to minimize the trauma to students and reduce the likelihood of copycat or further suicides (Leenaars and Wenckstern, 1998). School suicide postvention steps should include responding promptly after the event (within 24 hours of the suicide), acting in a concerned and conservative manner, informing all staff and school board members of the event and action steps, having teachers announce the death of the student to their first class of the day, making counseling sites available throughout the school, avoiding any glorification of the suicide, assigning a school liaison to handle media inquiries, monitoring the school's ongoing emotional climate, and evaluating all postvention activities (Goldeny and Berman, 1996; Peterson et al., 1993; NASB, 1998; Hassan, 1995; Roberts et al., 1998).

A major issue in suicide prevention programs is undiagnosed depression, including the reluctance of adolescents to report psychopathological symptoms to adults as well as to seek help from them

(Kalafat, 1997; Offer et al., 1991). In contrast, adolescents might be more inclined to report on their dissatisfaction with life to appropriate adults, thus serving as a proxy indicator for depression, suicide ideation or a potential suicide attempt. Ongoing monitoring of adolescents' life satisfaction reports could in part, promote the early identification of adolescents at risk for clinical depression, and perhaps eventual suicide ideation and behaviors (Frisch, 1998). In studies of adults, life dissatisfaction has been demonstrated to be an early sign of subsequent episodes of depression (Lesinsohn, Redner and Seeley, 1991). Similarly, adult life satisfaction has been related to the probability of relapses (Gonzales, Lewinsohn and Clark, 1985; Thunedborg et al., 1995). Interestingly, life satisfaction also influences the willingness of adults to participate in health promotion programs (Wagner et al., 1990). Given such findings, it seems worthwhile to explore the utility of adolescent life satisfaction reports as a component of suicide prevention programs.

CONCLUSIONS

It is difficult to explain from a cross-sectional study whether these adolescents reported suicide ideation or suicide behavior because of dissatisfaction with life or whether they are dissatisfied with life owing to suicide ideation and/or suicide behavior. Longitudinal, etiological and experimental studies are needed to determine whether dissatisfaction with life is a consequence or a determinant of suicide ideation/behavior. Nevertheless, this study revealed meaningful, robust relationships between perceived life dissatisfaction and self-reported poor mental health, suicide ideation and suicide behavior. In turn, effective suicide prevention programs should be structured enough to provide school professionals with guidelines to follow when dealing with this issue, yet flexible enough to allow for proper handling of unique situations.

ACKNOWLEDGMENTS

This research was funded by Cooperative Agreement #U63/CCU 802750–04, US Centers for Disease Control & Prevention, National

Center for Disease Prevention and Health Promotion, Division of Adolescent and School Health, Atlanta, Georgia, and Cooperative Agreements with the South Carolina Department of Education, Columbia, South Carolina.

REFERENCES

Andrews, F.M. and S.B. Withey: 1976, Social Indicators of Well-Being: Americans' Perceptions of Life Quality (Plenum, New York).

Brener, N.D., J.L. Collins, L. Kann, C.W. Warren and B.L. Williams: 1995, 'Reliability of the youth risk behavior survey questionnaire', American Journal of Epidemiology 141(6), pp. 575–580.

Capuzzi, D. and L. Golden: 1998, Preventing Adolescent Suicide (Accelerated Development, Inc., Muncie, IN).

Clark, D.B. and L. Kirisci: 1996, 'Postraumatic stress disorder, depression, alcohol use disorders and quality of life in adolescents', Anxiety 2, pp. 226–233.

Cochran, W.G.: 1963, Sampling Techniques, 2nd edition (John Wiley & Sons, New York), pp. 355–393.

Coker, A.L., R.E. McKeown, R.F. Valois and E.S. Huebner: 2000, 'Severe dating and violence, forced sex, and health-related quality of life among South Carolina high school students', American Journal of Preventive Medicine 19(4), pp. 1–10.

Compas, B: 1993, 'Promoting positive mental health in adolescence', in S.G. Millstein, A.C. Peterson and E.O. Nightingale (eds.), Promoting the Health of Adolescents (Oxford University Press, New York), pp. 159–179.

Day, H. and S.G. Jankey: 1996, 'Lessons from the literature: Toward a holistic model of quality of life', in R. Renwick, I. Brown and M. Nagler (eds.), Quality of Life in Health Promotion and Rehabilitation: Conceptual Approaches, Issues and Applications. (Sage, Thousand Oaks, CA), pp. 39–50.

Deiner, E.: 1994, 'Assessing subjective well-being: Progress and opportunities', Social Indicators Research 31, pp. 103–157.

Deiner, E.: 2000, 'Subjective well-being: the science of happiness and a proposal for a national index', American Psychologist 55, pp. 34–43.

Deiner, E., E. Suh, S. Oishi, R.E. Lucas and H.L. Smith: 1999, 'Subjective well-being: Three decades of progress', Psychological Bulletin 125, pp. 276–302.

Dew, T. and E.S. Huebner: 1994, 'Adolescent's perceived quality of life: An exploratory investigation', Journal of School psychology 32, pp. 185–199.

Dryfoos, J.G.: 1990, Adolescence at Risk: Prevalence and Prevention (Oxford University Press, New York), pp. 94–112.

DuRant, R.H., A.G. Getts, C. Cadenced, J. Emans and E.R. Woods: 1995, 'Exposure to violence and victimization and depression, hopelessness and purpose in life among adolescents living in or around public housing', Journal of Developmental Behavioral Pediatrics 16, pp. 233–237.

Federal Interagency Forum on Child and Family Statistics: 1997, 'America's children: Key national indicators of well-being' (Washington, DC).
Frisch, M.B.: 1998, 'Quality of life therapy and assessment in health care', Clinical Psychology: Science and Practice 5, pp. 19–40.
Frisch, M.N., J. Cornell, M. Villanueva and B. Retzlaff: 1992, 'Clinical validation of the quality of life inventory', Psychological Assessment 4, pp. 92–101.
Garrison, C.Z., R. McKeown, R.F. Valois and M.L. Vincent: 1993, 'Aggression, substance use, and suicidal behaviors in high school students', American Journal of Public Health 83(2), pp. 179–184.
Gilman, R. and E.S. Huebner: 1997, 'Children's reports of their life satisfaction: Convergence across raters, time and response formats', School Psychology International 18, pp. 133–147.
Gilman, R. and E.S. Huebner: 2000, 'Review of life satisfaction measures for adolescents', Behavior Change 17, pp. 178–183.
Gilman, R., E.S. Huebner and J.E. Laughlin: 2000, 'A first study of the multidimensional student life satisfaction scale with adolescents', Social Indicators Research 52, pp. 135–160.
Goldeny, R. and A. Berman: 1996, 'Postvention in schools: Affective or effective', Crisis 17(3), pp. 98–99.
Gonzales, L.R., P.M. Lewinsohn and G.N. Clark: 1985, 'Longitudinal follow-up of unipolar depressives: An investigation of predictors of relapse', Journal of Consulting and Clinical Psychology 53, pp. 461–469.
Hassan, R.: 1995, 'Effects of newspaper stories on the incidence of suicide in Australia: A research note', Australian and New Zealand Journal of Psychiatry 29(3), pp. 480–483.
Harris, E.C. and B. Barraclough: 1998, 'Excess mortality of mental disorders', British Journal of Psychiatry 173, pp. 11–53.
Headley B. and A. Wearing: 1989, 'Personality, life events and subjective well-being: Toward a dynamic equilibrium model', Journal of Personality and Social Psychology 57, pp. 731–739.
Hennessy, C.A., D.G. Morarity, M.M. Zack, P.A. Scherr and R. Brackbill: 1994, 'Measuring health-related quality of life for public health surveillance', Public Health Reports 109(5), pp. 665–672.
Hoyert, D.L., K.D. Kochanek and S.L. Murphy: 1999, 'Deaths: final data for 1997. National Center for Health Statistics', Monthly Vital Statistical Report 47(19), pp. 1–108.
Huebner, E.S.: 1991, 'Correlates of life satisfaction in children', School Psychology Quarterly 6, pp. 103–111.
Huebner, E.S.: 1997, 'Life satisfaction and happiness', in G. Bear, K. Minke and A. Thomas (eds.), Children's Needs II (National Association of School Psychologists, Silver Spring, MD), pp. 271–278.
Huebner, E.S. and G.L. Alderman: 1993, 'Convergent and discriminant validation of a children's life satisfaction scale: Its relationship to self- and teacher-reported psychological problems and school functioning', Social Indicators Research 30, pp. 71–82.

Huebner, E.S. and T. Dew: 1996, 'The interrelationships of positive affect, negative affect and life satisfaction in an adolescent sample', Social Indicators Research 38, pp. 129–137.

Huebner, E.S., J.W. Drane and R.F. Valois: 2000, 'Levels and demographic correlates of adolescent life satisfaction reports', School Psychology International 21(3), pp. 281–292.

Huebner, E.S., B.A. Funk and R. Gilman: 2000, 'Crosssectional and longitudinal psychosocial correlates of adolescent life satisfaction reports', Canadian Journal of School Psychology 16, pp. 53–64.

Huebner, E.S., J.E. Laughlin, C. Ash and R. Gilman: 1998, 'Further validation of the multidimensional students' satisfaction scale', Journal of Psychoeducational Assessment 16, pp. 118–134.

Huebner, E.S.: 1991, 'Initial development of the Students' Life Satisfaction Scale', School Psychology International 12, pp. 231–240.

Inglehart, R. and J.R. Rabier: 1986, 'Aspirations adapt to situation – but why are the Belgians so much happier than the French? A cross-cultural analysis of the subjective quality of life', in F.M. Andrews (ed.), Research on the Quality of Life (University of Michigan, Institute for Social Research, Ann Arbor MI), pp. 203–445.

Kalafat, J.: 1997, 'Prevention of youth suicide', in R. Weissberg, T. Gullotta, R. Hampton, B. Ryan & G. Adams (eds.), Enhancing Children's Wellness (Sage, Thousand Oaks, CA), pp. 175–213.

King, C.A.: 1997, 'Suicidal behavior in adolescence', in R.W. Maris, M.M. Silverman and S.S. Canetto (eds.), Review of Suicidology (Guliford Press, New York, NY), pp. 61–95.

King, K.A.: 2001, 'Developing a comprehensive school suicide prevention program', Journal of School Health 71(4), pp. 132–137.

Kolbe, L.J.: 1990, 'An epidemiological surveillance system to monitor the prevalence of youth behaviors that most affect health', Journal of Health Education 21(6), pp. 44–48.

Koivumaa-Honkanen, H., R. Honkanen, H. Viinamaki, K. Heikkila, J. Kaprio and M. Koskenvuo: 2001, 'Life satisfaction and suicide: A 20-year follow-up study', American Journal of Psychiatry 158(3), pp. 433–439.

Koivumaa-Honkanen, H., R. Honkanen, H. Viinamaki, K. Heikkila, J Kaprio and M. Koskenvuo: 2000, 'Self-reported life satisfaction and 20-Year mortality in healthy Finnish adults', American Journal of Epidemiology 152, pp. 983–991.

Koivumaa-Honkanen, H., H. Viinamaki, R. Honkanen, A. Tanskanen, R. Antikainen, L. Niskanen, J. Jaaskelainen and J. Lehtonen: 1996, 'Correlates of life satisfaction among psychiatric patients', Acta Psychiatry of Scandinavia 94, pp. 372–378.

Koivumaa-Honkanen, H., R. Honkanen, R. Antikainen, J. Hintikka and H. Viinamaki: 1999, 'Self-reported life satisfaction and treatment factors in patients with schizophrenia, major depression and anxiety disorder', Acta Psychiatry of Scandinavia 99, pp. 377–384.

Lazarus, R.: 1991, 'Progress on a cognitive-motivational-relational theory of emotion', American Psychologist 46, pp. 819–834.

Lester, D.: 1998, 'Life satisfaction, suicide, and homicide', Perceptual and Motor Skills 87, p. 126.

Leenaars, A.A. and S. Wenckstern: 1990, 'Post-traumatic stress disorder: A conceptual model for postvention', in A.A. Leenaars and S. Wenckstern (eds.), Suicide Prevention in the Schools (Hemisphere Publishing Corporation, New York, NY).

Leenaars, A.A. and S. Wenckstern: 1990, 'Principles of postvention: Applications to suicide and trauma in the schools', Death Studies 22(4), pp. 357–391.

McCullough, G., E.S. Huebner and J.E. Laughlin: 2000, 'Life events, self-concept and adolescents' positive subjective well-being,' Psychology in the School 37, pp. 281–290.

Morarity D. and M. Zack: 1999 'Validation of the US centers for disease control and prevention's healthy days measures' (abstract). Quality of Life Research Abstracts Issue, 6th Annual conference on the International Society of Quality of Life Research, Barcelona Spain 8(7), pp. 617.

Moscicki, E.K.: 1995, 'Epidemiology of suicidal behavior', Suicide and Life Threatening Behavior 25, pp. 22–35.

NASB-National School Boards Association: 1998, 'Suicide prevention', School Board News 18, p. 3.

Newcomb, M.D., P.M. Bentler and C. Collins: 1986, 'Alcohol use and dissatisfaction with self and life: A longitudinal analysis of young adults', Journal of Drug Issues 63, pp. 479–494.

Newschaffer, C.J.: 1998, Validation of the BRFSS HRQOL Measures in a Statewide Sample (US Department of Health and Human Services, Office of Disease Prevention and Health Promotion, Atlanta, 1997).

Offer, D., K.J. Howard, K.A. Schonert and E. Ostrov: 1991, 'To whom do adolescents turn for help? Differences between disturbed and nondistubed adolescents', Journal of the American Academy of Child & Adolescent Psychiatry 30, pp. 623–630.

Pavot, W., E. Diener, C.R. Colvin and E. Sandvik: 1991, 'Further validation of the satisfaction with Life Scale: evidence for the cross-method convergence of well being measures', Personality Assessment 57, pp. 149–161.

Peterson, B., P. Andress, L. Schrodeder, B. Swanson and L.M. Dolan-Ziff: 1993, 'The Edina, Minnesota, school crisis response team', Journal of School Health 63(4), pp. 192–193.

Raphael, D.: 1996, 'The determinants of adolescent health: Evolving definitions, recent findings, and proposed research agenda', Journal of Adolescent Health 9, pp. 6–16.

Raphael, D., E. Rukholm, I. Brown, P. Hill-Bailey and E. Donato: 1996, 'The Quality of Life Profile-Adolescent version: Background, description, and initial validation', Journal of Adolescent Health 7, pp. 366–375.

Renwick, R., I. Brown and N. Nagler (eds.): 1996, Quality of Life in Health Promotion and Rehabilitation: Conceptual Approaches, Issues and Applications (Sage, Thousand Oaks, CA).

Roberts, R.L., W.J. Lepowski and K.K. Davidson: 1998, 'Dealing with the aftermath of a student suicide: A T.E.A.M. approach', National Association of School Safety Bulletin 82, pp. 53–59.

Scales, P.C.: 1999, 'Reducing risks and building developmental assets: Essential actions for promoting adolescent health', Journal of School Health 69(3), pp. 113–119.

Seligman, M. and M. Csikszentmihalyi: 2000, 'Positive psychology: An introduction', American Psychologist 55, pp. 5–14.

Seligman, M.: 1998, 'What is the good life?' American Psychological Association Monitor 29(10), p. 2.

Seligson, J., E.S. Huebner and R.F. Valois: 2003, 'Preliminary validation of the Brief Multidimensional Student's Life Satisfaction Scale (BMSLSS)', Social Indicators Research 61, pp. 121–145.

Shah, B.V., B.G. Barnwell and G.S. Bieler: 1996, SUDAAN User's Manual, Release 7.0. Research Triangle Park (Research Triangle Institute, North Carolina).

Thatcher, W.G., B.M. Reininger and J.W. Drane: 2002, 'Using path analysis to examine adolescent suicide attempts, life satisfaction and health risk behavior', Journal of School Health 72(2), pp. 71–77.

Thunedborg, K., C.H. Black and P. Blech: 1995, 'Beyond the Hamilton Depression scores in long-term treatment of manic-melancholic patients: Prediction of recurrence of depression by quality of life instruments', Psychotherapy & Psychosomatics 64, pp. 131–140.

U.S. Department of Health & Human Services: 1991, Healthy People 2000: National Health Promotion and Disease Prevention Objectives (US Department of Health and Human Services, Washington, DC).

U.S. Public Health Service: 1999, Surgeon General's Call to Action of Prevent Suicide (U.S. Public Health Service, Washington, DC).

Valois, R.F. and T.B. Hoyle: 2000, 'Formative evaluation results of the Mariner Project: A coordinated school health pilot project', Journal of School Health 70(3), pp. 95–103.

Valois, R.F., M.L. Vincent, R. McKeown, C. Garrison and S. Kirby: 1993, 'Adolescent risk behaviors and the potential for violence: A look at what's coming to campus', American Journal of College Health 41(4), pp. 141–147.

Valois, R.F., K.J. Zullig and J.W. Drane: 2001 'Relationship between life satisfaction and violent behaviors among adolescents', American Journal of Health Behavior 25(4), pp. 353–366.

Valois, R.F., K.J. Zullig, E.S. Huebner, S.K. Kammermann and J.W. Drane: 2002, 'Relationship between of life satisfaction and sexual risk-taking behaviors among public high school adolescents', Journal of Child & Family Studies 11(4), pp. 427–440.

Veenhoven, R.: 1998, Bibliography of Happiness: 2472 Contemporary Studies of Subjective Appreciation in Life (RISBO, Rotterdam, Netherlands).

Wagner, E.H., V.J. Schoenbach, C.T. Orleans, L.C. Grothaus, K.W. Saunders, S. Curry and D.C. Pearson: 1990, 'Participation in a smoking cessation program: A population-based perspective', American Journal of Preventive Medicine 6, pp. 258–266.

Zullig, K.J., R.F. Valois, E.S. Huebner, J.W. Drane and J.E. Oeltmann: 2000, 'Relationship between selected substance abuse behaviors and adolescent self-perceptions of life satisfaction', Journal of Adolescent Health 29(4), pp. 1–11.

Zullig, K.J., R.F. Valois and J.W. Drane: 2002, 'Validity and reliability of the Health Related Quality of Life Health Days Measure for adolescents in a cross-section survey sample', Journal of Adolescent Health (Submitted for publication).

Health Promotion, Education & Behavior Robert F. Valois
Arnold School of Public Health
800 Sumter Street, Room 216
University of South Carolina
Columbia, SC 29208
USA
E-mail: RFValois@gwm.sc.edu

Department of Physical Education, Health & Sport Studies
Miami University Keith J. Zullig
Oxford, Ohio 45056
USA
E-mail: ZulligKJ@muohio.edu

Department of Psychology E. Scott Huebner
University of South Carolina
Columbia, SC 29208
USA
E-mail: Huebner@sc.edu

Epidemiology & Biostatistics J. Wanzer Drane
Arnold School of Public Health
800 Sumter Street, Room 202
University of South Carolina
Columbia, SC 29208
USA
E-mail: Wdrane@gwm.sc.edu

KAREN MARRIAGE and ROBERT A. CUMMINS

SUBJECTIVE QUALITY OF LIFE AND SELF-ESTEEM IN CHILDREN: THE ROLE OF PRIMARY AND SECONDARY CONTROL IN COPING WITH EVERYDAY STRESS

ABSTRACT. Two major predictors of subjective quality of life (SQOL) in adults are known to be self-esteem and a sense of primary control. Moreover, secondary control is known to be an important defence strategy when primary control fails. This study aimed to determine whether these relationships also apply to children. A sample of 66 children aged from 5 to 12 years were compared on their use of primary and secondary control and on their ratings of SQOL and self-esteem. SQOL was measured using the Comprehensive Quality of Life Scale, self-esteem by using the Coopersmith Self-Esteem Inventory, and primary and secondary control were measured by coding children's responses to three short video clips of children in stressful situations. It was found that younger children use more primary control and less secondary control than older children. However, five year olds were found capable of producing secondary control strategies. Contrary to expectation, primary and secondary control did not predict either self-esteem or SQOL. However, self-esteem predicted SQOL as expected and no sex differences were found. These findings emphasise important differences from the adult literature and the reasons for this are discussed.

Satisfaction with Life and Self

Childhood is said to be the happiest time of life but the question of just how happy children are, and why, has received little research attention. This is in contrast to research on adults where much recent progress has been made in understanding the normative level of subjective quality of life (SQOL). In particular, while it has been known for some time that SQOL tends to evidence fairly high levels of positivity (Headey and Wearing, 1992), more recent evidence has indicated a remarkable level of consistency. A series of reports (Cummins, 1995, 1996, 1998) has revealed that, if Likert scale data are recoded to a 0–100 scale, the mean population level of life satisfaction can be expressed as 75 ± 2.5. The values that result from this recoding procedure are expressed in units called 'percentage of scale maximum' (%SM). Thus, using two standard deviations to

Social Indicators Research **66:** 107–122, 2004.

define a normal distribution, the mean score of normative population samples predictably lies within the range of 70–80%SM. This level of consistency has led to the hypothesis that SQOL may be held under homeostatic control, and empirical evidence for this has been provided (Cummins, 2000a, 2003). However, whether such consistency applied to children is not known.

Research into the SQOL of children has been hampered by various issues. For example, most studies have been conducted using disadvantaged or physically ill children, limiting what we know of the normative course of well-being. Moreover, most studies do not ask children to comment on their own perceptions of well-being. Instead they rely on objective measures such as educational achievement or psychopathology (e.g., Nespoli et al., 1995), or on the report of a third party responding for the child (e.g., Hoare, 1993). This latter technique is now known to be invalid in relation to the self-perceptions of the individual concerned (Cummins, 2002). So, a major problem is instrumentation. New instruments are required that do not require advanced cognitive and language skills, and yet are able to measure SQOL by children's self reports. These difficulties have already been tackled in the quality of life literature pertaining to adults who are intellectually or cognitively disabled. The Comprehensive Quality of Life Scale – Adult, Fifth Edition (ComQol-A5; Cummins, 1997a) has a parallel version for this purpose (ComQol-I5; Cummins, 1997b). As with the original adult scale, this measure asks respondents to indicate their satisfaction with a number of life domains and to rate the degree to which each life domain is important to them. This scale is completed by pointing to a series of pictures. Due to the simplicity of ComQol-I5 and its ability to be used by people of varying cognitive capacities, one aim of the current study is to determine whether this version of the scale may also be used with children.

Control and Satisfaction with the Self

A recently published model concerning the psychological processes responsible for generating SQOL has emphasised the importance of self-esteem and control (Cummins, 2000b). While the link with self-esteem is now thoroughly documented (see, e.g., Diener and Diener, 1995), literature concerning the link between SQOL and control is more diverse. This is due, in no small part, to the lack of any agreed definition of perceived control.

One recent formulation that is gathering increasing research attention involves the description of control as Primary and Secondary (Rothbaum et al., 1982; Heckhausen and Schulz, 1993). In this scheme primary control reflects control over the existing physical, social or behavioural realities, while secondary control reflects internal control of the self in situations where primary control either is not, or cannot, be exercised. Thus, in Western societies at least, primary control is generally seen as the preferred strategy, with secondary control used to reduce the negative psychological impact of uncontrollable objective conditions or events (Band and Weisz, 1990).

In confirmation of this description, several studies have found positive correlations between primary control and subjective well-being (e.g., Schulz and Decker, 1985) and happiness (e.g., Larson, 1989). However, the empirical demonstration of the role of secondary control in this regard is less certain, most particularly in relation to children.

The Development of Control in Children

Although much is known about how children respond to highly stressful and traumatic situations, such as the death of a parent (e.g., Felner et al., 1981) or divorce (e.g., Hetherington, 1984), there is a relative paucity of research into how children respond to everyday stressful events. Further, it is unclear whether children's use of primary and secondary control impacts upon their self-esteem and perceived well-being in the same way as adults.

A complicating factor is that each form of control emerges at different points in development. While primary control strategies are present from birth (Heckhausen and Schulz, 1995) (e.g., when an infant cries when hungry) secondary control seems to emerge at a later age with a time course that is at yet uncertain. Certainly most authors agree that the use of secondary control increases throughout middle childhood (e.g., Altshuler and Ruble, 1989; Band and Weisz, 1990; Compas et al., 1991; Heckhausen and Schulz, 1995) but the age at which secondary control emerges as a functional psychological device is not known. While Altshuler and Ruble (1989) demonstrated that children as young as five or six have some limited experience of the secondary control processes of cognitive and behavioural distraction, the use of other secondary control strategies at such a young age remains undetermined. Thus, it is unclear at what age the use of primary and secondary control begins to resemble that used by adults.

This study will measure primary and secondary control in children between the ages of five and 12 to determine the development of these styles of coping and whether secondary control is present in 5 year-olds. It will also examine whether the control strategies used by children are associated with SQOL and self-esteem.

METHOD

Participants

The study involved 66 children recruited from three public primary schools in the North, North-West and Eastern suburbs of Melbourne. The participants ranged in age from five to 12 years, with an average age of 8.5 ± 2.1 years and 45.5 percent were female. The parents of all children in each class were asked to allow their child to participate and the average rate of consent was 21% across the schools. Each approved child was also asked to consent to participate and told that they were free to withdraw at any time. One child refused to participate.

Materials

Data were collected using two scales and responses to videotaped scenarios. The scale used to measure SQOL was the intellectual/cognitive disability version of the Comprehensive Quality of Life Scale (ComQol-I5; Cummins, 1997b). The subjective component of this scale utilises two sub-scales that measure the satisfaction with, and the importance of, seven domains of life. These domains are, in order, material well-being, health, productivity, relationships (here separated into relationships with friends and relationship with family), safety, place in community, and emotional well-being. Satisfaction is recorded by pointing to a set of five faces ranging from very sad to very happy. Importance is recorded by pointing to a series of drawings with children standing on five steps increasing in height, with the posture and expression of each child indicating the relative level of importance. ComQol-I5 has been demonstrated to be reliable, stable, valid and sensitive when used with an intellectually disabled population (Cummins, 1999) although this scale is yet to be used with children. The scale can be accessed through the web-site http://acqol.deakin.edu.au or by writing to the second author.

The Coopersmith Self Esteem inventory (School Form, Coopersmith, 1981) is a standardised scale to measure self esteem among children. It contains 58 items that are responded to with "like me" or "not like me" answers. These items comprise four subscales; general self esteem (e.g., things usually don't bother me), social self esteem (e.g., I'm popular with kids my own age), home esteem (e.g., my parents usually consider my feelings) and school esteem (e.g., I am proud of my school work), and a lie scale (e.g., I like everyone I know).

In order to measure primary, secondary and relinquished control, a number of one minute duration video tapes were prepared. Each video depicted an everyday stressful situation being experienced by a child. The scenarios were taken from several used by Band and Weisz (1988) and covered the situations of "another child saying something mean" (containing two children sitting in the playground talking. For example "I don't want to be your best friend, your secrets are just boring, that's why nobody likes you"), "going to the doctor to get a needle" (set in the doctors surgery with the doctor drawing up a syringe and asking the child to pull up their sleeve) and "falling over, spilling hot chips and getting hurt" (in which a child buys a bag of hot chips but drops them due to tripping over a school bag). Only these three scenarios were chosen from the six used by Band and Weisz (1988) due to ease of scripting and as all but the medical situation were found by these authors to elicit similar responses.

A professional script developer, camera operator, sound recorder and actors were engaged in the production of these videos. Each of the three chosen scenarios was filmed four times, once with female aged between six and seven, once with female actors aged between

10 and 11, once with male actors aged between six and seven and finally with male actors aged between 10 and 11. A copy of these tapes is available from the second author.

In the administration of these videos, each participant watched the video corresponding to their sex and closest to their age. The order in which the three scenarios were presented was counterbalanced. A fourth scenario was viewed by each participant at the completion of testing, depicting the happy situation of a child receiving a present in the mail, to ensure that children left the testing situation in a positive frame of mind. No data were recorded for this scenario.

Procedure

Approval from the Deakin University Ethics Committee and the Department of Education was obtained prior to commencement of this study.

Although ComQol-I5 has provision for respondents to use a two or three point scale, initial pilot testing with five year old children indicated that they were able to reliably respond to five-point scales that were pictorially represented. They were also able to respond to the self esteem questionnaire when it was orally presented. Participants aged between five and eight years of age were interviewed individually and their answers were recorded verbatim by the investigator. Children aged over eight were interviewed in pairs and wrote their own answers on record sheets. All children had the items read aloud to them. The interviews took place in a quiet room away from the classroom.

Participants initially provided their age which was verified using school records. Each child completed the subjective component of ComQol-I5, then the Coopersmith Self Esteem Inventory and then watched the three target video scenes followed by the happy scene. For the three target scenarios each child was asked by the investigator: "how do you think this boy/girl is feeling?", and "what could he/she do or think to make it feel better?". To assess the underlying goal of the strategy given they were asked "and how do you think that would help to make it feel better?" Children were then asked "If they couldn't do/think ____, what else could they do or think to make it feel better?" This was again followed by the question "and how do you think that ____ would help to make it feel better?" to assess the underlying goal of the strategy. Although some variation in questioning was inevitable during the interview, the questions were administered as uniformly as possible to minimise differential social cues. Further, each child was either interviewed individually or, when interviewed in pairs, wrote their own answers, thus ensuring the confidentiality of their responses.

Data Coding

Each response to the videotape scenarios was coded as being one of primary, secondary or relinquished control following the system described by Band and Weisz (1988). Responses were coded as primary control when the action was directed at modifying or influencing circumstances, events, objects or other people so as to enhance rewards by bringing objective conditions into line with the wishes of the child. For example "he should pick up the chips and eat them anyway and then he won't care about it" or "go and tell the teacher. She'll make him apologise for being so mean".

Responses were coded as secondary control when efforts were made to modify or influence the child's subjective psychological state (e.g., their wishes, expectations, mood, attributions, interpretations) so as to enhance rewards by achieving comfortable accommodation, or goodness of fit with respect to conditions as they are. For example, in response to the scenario of another child saying something mean, a secondary control response might be "she should do her favourite things, it would take her mind off it" or, to the getting a needle scenario "think about something happy, it would distract her from the needle".

Responses were coded as relinquished control when the response both failed to enhance reward or reduce punishment, and implied passive acceptance. For example, "there is nothing that she could do" or "she would just have to put up with it".

Table I indicates examples of responses coded as Primary and Secondary control. These have been arranged corresponding to the three scenes.

Inter-rater reliability for the primary-secondary-relinquished control coding was assessed by having two raters independently judge 90 responses from 15 randomly selected children. Raters were

TABLE I

Sample primary and secondary control responses for each scenario

Scenario title	Primary control responses	Secondary control responses
A child says something mean	Go and find another friend to play with.	Just ignore her.
	Get the teacher to make him be nice to you.	Remember that you've got other friends to play with.
Going to the doctors for a needle	Run out of the room.	Think of happy thoughts.
	Hold your breath to stop the pain.	Look away.
Falling over	Go and buy some more chips.	Try not to think about it.
	Get a bandage from your mum.	Don't let yourself worry about, just be happy.

blind to the subject's age and sex. Reliability analysis yielded a pairwise kappa value of 0.88.

RESULTS

Prior to analysis, all variables were screened for normality, linearity, and univariate outliers. Sixteen participants were unable to provide answers for some of the six control questions producing a total of 19 missing data points. These individual responses were excluded from the analyses, and the cases retained. SQOL and self esteem data, being naturally negatively skewed were not transformed (Tabachnick and Fidell, 1989).

The first form of analysis involved the calculation of reliability coefficients for ComQol-I5 to assess its use with children. The reliability (Cronbach's alpha) of the importance subscale was 0.66, of the satisfaction subscale was 0.58, and of the combined SQOL score was 0.64. These scores are consistent with data reported by Cummins (1997b) regarding the use of the scale with an adult population with an intellectual disability and are within the acceptable range for internal consistency suggested by Boyle (1991). Two other aspects of the data are notable. First that the mean scores fall into the normative range 70–80%SM range established for adults

TABLE II

Means and standard deviations (SD) for self esteem, primary, secondary and relinquished control, and SQOL (SWB) for younger and older children

Variable	Younger		Older	
	Mean	SD	Mean	SD
Primary control	57.48	25.32	41.65	26.66
Secondary control	27.82	19.99	54.98	27.16
Relinquished control	2.99	9.33	2.33	7.50
SQOL material	71.05	26.72	78.10	19.83
SQOL health	78.53	22.37	71.10	25.63
SQOL productivity	77.77	18.58	72.70	12.27
SQOL friend	74.65	28.06	92.67	12.12
SQOL family	81.61	28.51	92.62	13.19
SQOL safety	77.63	26.41	71.81	29.25
SQOL community	52.25	29.57	72.27	17.05
SQOL emotion	86.32	17.50	80.31	22.75
Total SQOL	74.98	13.91	78.95	10.24
Self esteem	66.37	15.62	70.18	15.74

The SQOL scores presented in this paper have been converted to a percentage of scale maximum (%SM) score, as if the scoring was from 0–100.

(Table II). Second, that the distinctive domain pattern of high scores on family and low on community, characteristic of normal adult data (Cummins, 1997a) are also evident here. It would thus appear that the ComQol-I5 exhibits similar psychometric characteristics when used with children as it does with adults.

Table III examines the sequence of the first two control responses provided by five year old children (n = 7), six to eight year old children (n = 31) and nine to 12 year old children (n = 28) in the three stressful scenarios. The responses of the five year olds are displayed alone to emphasise the response patterns in the youngest children. Age groupings were chosen to demonstrate age related changes that took place in the use of primary and secondary control.

This table indicates that, in scenario 1 there are clear age-related differences, with younger children providing greater numbers of primary control responses and fewer secondary control responses

TABLE III

Frequency of control response patterns

Age	Scenario#	Control response sequence			
		P/P*	P/S	S/P	S/S
5 yr olds	1	60.0	20.0	0	20.0
5 yr olds	2	66.6	12.5	0	33.3
5 yr olds	3	66.6	16.6	0	16.6
6–8	1	58.3	16.6	12.5	12.5
6–8	2	37.5	20.8	4.2	37.5
6–8	3	61.3	9.7	9.7	19.4
9–12	1	38.5	30.8	7.7	23.1
9–12	2	3.9	11.5	7.7	76.9
9–12	3	63.2	0	26.3	26.3

#Scenario 1 = another child saying something mean; Scenario 2 = going to the doctor to get a needle; Scenario 3 = falling over, dropping your chips and hurting your knee.
*P = Primary control response; S = Secondary control response.

than older children. Scenario 2 was more likely than other scenarios to evoke secondary control responses in all age groups and it provided the clearest indication of age related changes. Overall it can be seen that primary control responses are more common than secondary control responses and that children most commonly provide both answers within the one control category (for example primary control followed by another primary control response). Children as young as five are able to provide secondary control responses in all three scenarios and, interestingly, five year olds did not answer with the secondary control followed by primary control pattern. In summary, it appears that children respond with different coping strategies in different scenarios and that there are clear age-related changes in the coping strategies chosen.

To test the hypotheses that younger children will use more primary control strategies and older children will use more secondary control strategies a Multivariate Analysis of Variance was performed. Pillai's criterion was significant as $F(1, 642) = 8.84$, ($p < 0.001$). Results of the univariate F-tests for significant with

TABLE IV

Univariate comparisons for younger and older children on primary and secondary control

Dependent variables	F	P<	Younger	Older
			Mean (SD)	Mean (SD)
Primary control	6.33	0.01	57.81 (25.32)	41.65 (26.66)
Secondary control	22.00	0.001	27.83 (19.99)	54.81 (27.16)
Relinquished control	0.10	NS	2.99 (9.32)	2.33 (7.50)

TABLE V

Standard multiple regression analysis with self esteem, primary control and secondary control as predictors of SQOL

Variable	SQOL (DV)	PC	SC	B	(ß)	Sr^2 unique
Primary control	–0.01			1.29	0.16	0.01
Secondary control	0.15	–0.77		1.93	0.24	0.02
Self esteem	0.42	0.02	0.08	0.32	0.39	0.15*
				$R^2 = 0.20^{\#}$		
				Adjusted $R^2 = 0.17$		

#Unique variability = 0.18; Shared variability = 0.02.
*$p < 0.01$.

the means and standard deviations for children aged 5–8 and 9–12 are presented in Table IV. It can be seen that the younger children used significantly more primary control and less secondary control than older children.

To test the hypotheses that self esteem, primary and secondary control will predict SQOL, a standard multiple regression analysis was performed and is presented in Table V. R for regression was significantly different from zero, $F(3, 62) = 5.27$, $p < 0.05$, and the combination of independent variables predicted 20 percent (17 percent adjusted) of the variability in SQOL. However, self esteem was the only significant predictor, explaining 15 percent of the variability in SQOL. Because neither of the control variables significantly predicted SQOL the hypothesis was only partially supported.

Two final exploratory analyses were conducted. The first involved a standard regression to determined the extent to which primary and secondary control predict self esteem. This was found not to be significant. The second employed a multivariate analysis of variance to determine whether there are sex differences in SWB, self esteem, primary and secondary or relinquished control. Again, no significance was found. In summary, ComQol-I5 was found to be a reliable measure of SQOL in children, with children reporting similarly high levels of SQOL to that of adults. It was also found that while younger children use more primary control and less secondary control than older children, even five year olds were capable of producing secondary control strategies. However, the type of stressful event influenced the type of control strategy chosen by children. Surprisingly, neither primary nor secondary control predicted self esteem or SQOL, although self esteem was found to predict SQOL. No sex differences were found in the data.

DISCUSSION

The most interesting finding from this investigation is that children aged five years are able to apply secondary control strategies to vicarious scenarios depicting an acute loss of primary control. Certainly the frequency with which these children volunteered secondary control strategies was less than the frequency for older children. But these data extend the known age at which children are capable of generating such cognitive devices.

The most likely explanation for the increase in secondary control with age is as a function of cognitive maturation. As suggested by Band (1990) secondary control would be expected to increase as children learn that there is much about the world that is beyond their control and thus develop secondary control as a buffer to negative affect in these circumstances.

However, in contrast to the findings of Band (1990) and Band and Weisz (1990) we did not find that children of all ages use more primary than secondary control. Rather, it was found that secondary control became the favoured control strategy of older children. This discrepancy is possibly due to the different samples and type of stress utilised in the design of the studies. In the 1990 studies, the samples consisted of children with diabetes who were asked about how they coped with their illness. It is possible that both younger and older children in these studies continued to use predominantly primary control strategies, such as taking medication or monitoring diet, as these behaviours are crucial to their continued health. The present study, on the other hand, used children from the general population and scenarios with less serious consequences for non-primary control responses.

Children's preferred styles of coping also differed depending upon the type of situation with which they were presented. Consistent with the findings of Band and Weisz (1988) it was found that children reported substantially more primary control in the peer difficulty and physical accident situations than in the medical procedure situation in which they were far more likely to use secondary control. This pattern was observed across all age groups. It is possible that the children viewed the medical situation as less controllable and found it necessary to use approaches that aimed at controlling the psychological impact of the stress of getting a needle. In contrast, being rejected by a peer or falling over may be more familiar to a child and they may have practiced successful ways to modify such objective circumstances and outcomes.

It is interesting that these preferred control strategies did not predict SQOL or self esteem. This finding differs from those obtained by Petito (1998) who found both primary and secondary control to predict well-being in a sample of adolescents. While both studies used similar methods to establish well-being, they differed in their measurement of primary and secondary control. The Petito study used conventional questionnaire techniques, compared with the control scenario techniques used here. It is therefore possible that the similarity in method of data collection in the previous study facilitated shared variance between the measured variables. Alternatively, the measurement of control through video clips may not provide a reliable estimate of more generalized response tendencies. These possibilities require further investigation.

Another important finding for future research was that the ComQol-I5 appeared to be quite suitable for use with children. In terms of reliability it produced comparable internal reliability and pattern of domain data to adults. This suggests that ComQol-I5 is a reliable measure of SQOL in children. Moreover, it appears to be valid as judged by the group mean of 76.7%SM lying well within the normative adult range of 70–80%SM (Cummins, 1995, 1998), and the standard deviation of 12.6%SM is also equivalent to that obtained with adult samples.

In terms of ComQol sensitivity, differences were apparent between the domain ratings of younger (under 9 years) and older (over 9 years) children. A large discrepancy between the groups was found in the life domain of place in the community, which young children rated lowest. This may be explained by the limited social experience that very young children have outside the home and school. Younger children also rated the closeness to friends substantially lower than did the older children who may have begun to realise the importance of social support. Further younger children rated higher well-being scores on the domain of family than friends, perhaps indicating the greater amount of emphasis that family plays in the lives of younger children.

Finally, despite these domain based differences, no sex differences were found in SQOL. This finding is consistent with a large adult literature (e.g., Collette, 1984; Liang, 1984) which finds both adult males and females to be similarly satisfied with their lives. Thus it appears that this similarity is present even in children as young as five years of age.

In conclusion it appears that ComQol-I5 is a reliable, valid and sensitive measure of SQOL for children as young as five years. It has also been determined that children as young as five years of age are capable of using secondary control strategies. Moreover, the increasing use of such strategies with age is consistent with expectation and evidence of methodological validity. It is therefore of some interest that neither primary nor secondary control correlated with SQOL or self-esteem. This finding was unexpected and may indicate method effects which deserve further investigation.

REFERENCES

Altshuler, J.L. and D.N. Ruble: 1989, 'Developmental changes in children's awareness of strategies for coping with uncontrollable stress', Child Development 60, pp. 1337–1349.

Band, E.B.: 1990, 'Children's coping with diabetes: Understanding the role of cognitive development', Journal of Pediatric Psychology 15, pp. 27–41.
Band, E.B. and J.R. Weisz: 1988, 'How to feel better when it feels bad: Children's perspectives on coping with everyday stress', Developmental Psychology 24, pp. 247–253.
Band, E.B. and J.R. Weisz: 1990, 'Developmental differences in primary and secondary control coping and adjustment to juvenile diabetes', Journal of Clinical Child Psychology 19, pp. 150–158.
Boyle, G.J.: 1991, 'Does item homogeneity indicate internal consistency of item redundancy in psychometric scales?', Personality and Individual Differences 12, pp. 291–294.
Collette, J.: 1984, 'Sex differences in life satisfaction: Australian data', Journal of Gerontology 39, pp. 243–245.
Compas, B.E., G.A. Bancz, V. Maleame and N. Worsham: 1991, 'Perceived control and coping with stress: A developmental perspective', Journal of Social Issues 47, pp. 23–34.
Coopersmith, S.: 1981, Coopersmith Self Esteem Inventories (Consulting Psychologists Press Inc., California).
Cummins, R.A.: 1995, 'On the trail of the gold-standard for SQOL', Social Indicators Research 35, pp. 179–200.
Cummins, R.A.: 1996, 'The domains of life satisfaction: An attempt to order chaos', Social Indicators Research 38, pp. 303–332.
Cummins, R.A.: 1997a, Comprehensive Quality of Life Scale-Adult: ComOol-A5, 5th ed. (School Of Psychology, Deakin University, Melbourne).
Cummins, R.A.: 1997b, Comprehensive Quality of Life Scale-Intellectual/Cognitive Disability: ComQol-I5, 5th edition (School Of Psychology, Deakin University, Melbourne).
Cummins, R.A.: 1998, 'The second approximation to an international standard of life satisfaction', Social Indicators Research 43, pp. 307–334.
Cummins, R.A.: (1999), 'A psychometric evaluation of the Comprehensive Quality of Life Scale', in L.L. Yuan, B. Yuen and C. Low (eds.), Urban Quality of Life: Critical Issues and Options, 5th ed. (National University of Singapore, Singapore), pp. 32–46.
Cummins, R.A.: 2000a, 'A homeostatic model for subjective quality of life', Proceedings, Second Conference of Quality of Life in Cities (National University of Singapore, Singapore), pp. 51–59.
Cummins, R.A.: 2000b, 'Personal income and subjective well-being: A review', Journal of Happiness Studies 1, pp. 133–158.
Cummins, R.A.: 2002, 'Proxy responding for subjective well-being: A review', International Review of Research in Mental Retardation 25, pp. 183–207.
Cummins, R.A.: 2003, 'Normative life satisfaction: Measurement issues and a homeostatic model', Social Indicators Research (in press).
Diener, E. and M. Diener: 1995, 'Cross-cultural correlates of life satisfaction and self esteem', Journal of Personality and Social Psychology 68, pp. 653–663.

Felner, R.D., M.A. Ginter, M.F. Boike and E.L. Cowen: 1981, 'Parental death or divorce and the school adjustment of young children', American Journal of Community Psychology 9, pp. 181–191.

Headey, B. and A. Wearing: 1992, Understanding Happiness: A Theory of Subjective Well-being (Longman Cheshire, Melbourne).

Heckhausen, J. and R. Schulz: 1993, 'Optimisation by selection and compensation: Balancing primary and secondary control in the life span development', International Journal of Behavioral Development 16, pp. 287–303.

Heckhausen, J. and R. Schulz: 1995, 'A life-span theory of control', Psychological Bulletin 102, pp. 284–304.

Hetherington, M.E.: 1984, 'Stress and coping in children and families', New Directions for Child Development 24, pp. 7–33.

Hoare, P.: 1993, 'The quality of life of children with chronic epilepsy and their families', Seizure 2, pp. 269–275.

Larson, R.: 1989, 'Is feeling 'in control' related to happiness in daily life?', Psychological Reports 64, pp. 775–784.

Liang, J.: 1984, 'Dimensions of the satisfaction with life index: A structural formulation', Journal of Gerontology 39, pp. 613–622.

Nespoli, L., A.P. Verri, F. Locatelli, L. Bertuggia, R.M. Taibi and G.R. Burgio: 1995, 'The impact of paediatric bone marrow transplantation on quality of life', Quality of Life Research 4, pp. 233–240.

Petito, F.: 1998, 'An evaluation of primary and secondary control processes on the subjective quality of life of adolescents', unpublished masters thesis, Deakin University.

Rothbaum, F., J.R. Weisz and S.S. Snyder: 1982, 'Changing the world and changing the self. A two-process model of perceived control', Journal of Personality and Social Psychology 42, pp. 5–37.

Schulz, R. and S. Decker: 1985, 'Long-term adjustment to physical disability: The role of social support, perceived control, and self blame', Journal of Personality and Social Psychology 48, pp. 1162–1172.

Tabachnick, B.G. and L.S. Fidell: 1989, Using Multivariate Statistics, 2nd ed. (Harper and Row Publishers, New York).

School of Psychology
Deakin University
221 Burwood Hwy
Burwood, Victoria 3125
Australia
E-mail: cummins@deakin.edu.au

FERRAN CASAS, MÒNICA GONZÁLEZ, CRISTINA FIGUER and GERMÀ COENDERS

SUBJECTIVE WELL-BEING, VALUES AND GOAL ACHIEVEMENT

ABSTRACT. The relation between life domains satisfaction and overall life satisfaction, values, internal/external perceived control and the option of planning or by chance searching information on the Internet has been explored in a sample of Spanish adolescents aged 12 to 16 (N=968). Age and sex differences have been examined. Results clearly confirm a positive relation between satisfaction with life domains and overall satisfaction with life. Satisfaction with life as a whole shows also to be positively correlated with non-materialistic values. Perceived control shows to be, once again, a key construct to understand both life-satisfaction of adolescents and their behavioural intentions to plan or not to plan their action to fulfil intended goals. A clear pattern between external and internal perceived control stems from our analysis: subjects reporting to rely on chance when searching information show higher external perceived control while respondents who prefer to plan show higher internal perceived control. The more satisfaction expressed with learning related items (satisfaction with school performance, learning, and preparation for future), with family and with life as a whole, the more tendencies are observed among the respondents to plan their search. No direct relation has been observed between values and behavioural intentions to plan or not to plan action to fulfil intended goals. Perceived control, but also satisfaction with some life domains and with life as a whole seem to act as mediating factors between behavioural intentions and values.

KEY WORDS: by chance, children, goal achievement, Internet, life-satisfaction, perceived control, plan, values

INTRODUCTION

Relationship between goal achievement behaviours and subjective quality of life has not been explored very often among adolescents. Goal achievement is one of human behaviours related to aspirations. From the point of view of Campbell et al. (1976) quality of life studies should consider not only perceptions and evaluations,

Social Indicators Research **66:** 123–141, 2004.

but also aspirations of people. Aspirations are a complex concept and social sciences have not yet developed many debates about theoretical models and procedures to get good measures of people's aspirations in different contexts.

We may consider aspirations at least at two very different levels:

(a) General aspirations, which are usually formulated in abstract terms. General aspirations, particularly among pedagogues, have often been related to values, i.e.: values the subject aspirates to be appreciated for, in his or her future life. In any case, in our present research we are interested in aspirations as conscious goals of people, not as just dreams.
(b) Concrete aspirations, which are often related to concrete goals the subject wants to achieve, at his or her present period of life.

On the other hand, as many authors have yet pointed out, for the last decade an important number of studies on children's subjective well-being has been published, although this field of study is still in its infancy if compared with adult's SWB studies (Huebner, 1994; Casas et al., 2001). Such studies have often tested measures of how children and adolescents evaluate their overall life satisfaction and their satisfaction with specific domains of life. However, we have not been able to find much research of under 16's in which life satisfaction is studied in relation to life general aspirations, as for example, values. In fact, we have found more scientific literature analysing the relationship between the own value system and planning strategies to reach own goals, than analysing the relation between subjective well-being and values.

Field observation has repeatedly suggested that children feel happy when they perceive they have active influence in the process of reaching goals related to concrete aspirations (Hart, 1992). However, the existence of an aspiration, obviously, does not imply there will be a proactive attitude to get this aspiration to become reality. In real life, people have to decide whether they want to plan concrete actions to fulfil their goals, or not (Friedman et al., 1987).

Under which conditions individuals decide to plan how to reach the fulfilment of general or concrete aspirations? Does life satisfaction have any influence on this decision to plan or not?

Such questions are very important and, in fact, answers to the first one have often been explored among adolescents in relation to behaviours such as, for example, avoiding an undesired pregnancy or finding a concrete kind of job to get money (Friedman and Scholnick, 1997; Martin et al., 1998).

Different authors underline that necessary preconditions to decide to plan the achievement of concrete goals are that the individual has to believe that planning is important and that the goal toward which planning is directed is important (Nurmi, 1993). Judgements about what is important, according to other authors are closely linked to the individuals' value system (Kreiter and Kreiter, 1987). In any case, there is certain agreement that environments, beliefs, values and practices are factors that have influence on the fact of planning (Friedman and Scholnick, 1997). And some authors also emphasize that another precondition to plan is that individuals believe in their capacity as planners and as implementers of the particular strategy generated (Skinner and Connel, 1986; Nurmi, 1991), as for example, because they have appropriated preparation or skills.

Social psychologists have defined values as preferential frameworks to guide individual behaviours in the world that can only be understood in the context of social interactions (Garzón and Garcés, 1989). Often beliefs and value systems have a hierarchical structure, some of them being more nuclear than other (Rokeach, 1973). Although the value system of each individual is pretty stable, it may change in different social contexts and in different cultural conditions, and it is particularly influenced by social and political development of each society (Pinillos, 1982).

The relation between values of children and SWB seems to be potentially able to raise rather new debates. Do adolescents high in materialistic values tend to be more or less satisfied with life than those high in more humanistic values? Or perhaps values make no big differences in people's life satisfaction? Does the fact of being satisfied with life or with a specific life domain have any relation with different aspirated values?

Such discussion cannot ignore the old psychosocial research tradition that has produced an extensive literature relating the *locus control* with the kind of attributions made by people. According to such tradition it seems obvious we should hypothesise that external or internal perceived control is related to passive or proactive attitudes towards working for own aspirations. In fact, according to Skinner (1997), perceived control is no longer considered a stable personality factor, but rather a *set of beliefs* that children and adults hold about how the causal world works and about their individual role in producing desired events in their own lives. On the other hand, perceived control, together with self-esteem and other internal personality variables have often been identified as correlated with satisfaction among children and adolescents (Huebner, 1991; Huebner and Dew, 1993).

We know that some people plan actively the fulfilment of their goals and some other people remain rather passive, expecting that others or perhaps serendipity will help. To what extent is that attitude related to life satisfaction, or is life satisfaction influenced by such attitude?

We have raised a set of important questions in this introductory statement. We do not intend to give a unique and clear answer to such important questions with this preliminary research. However, we intend to make some contribution in order to propose directions and challenges to go on researching. One of our basic hypotheses is that aspirations – both concrete aspirations and aspirated values – and subjective well-being of children are related in some way or another. Our aim is to explore the relationships among factors involved in the process of fulfilling goals related to concrete aspirations, i.e.: subjective well-being, values, perceived control, and the option of planning or searching by chance.

Taking into account that most children need to explain their action strategies in very concrete – non abstract – situations, we decided to explore children's strategic options when looking for something in a concrete medium – highly motivating for them – as the Internet.

All of these introductory considerations brought us to design our study with the purpose of analysing possible relationships among constructs displayed in the boxes in Figure 1.

METHOD

Procedure and Sample

Data from this study were obtained by administering a questionnaire to students in compulsory secondary education in Catalonia (N.E. of Spain), aged 12 to 16 years old. Children belonged to

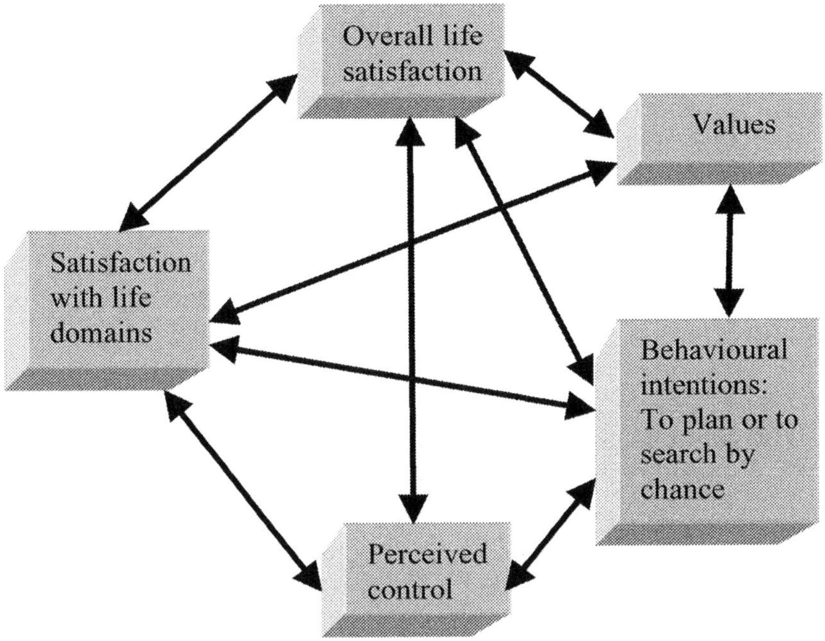

Figure 1. Hypothetical relationships among constructs explored in this study.

an intentional selection of classrooms by school, planned in order to get a sample of middle class students attending regular schools that were considered to have a population of students illustrative of the most frequent characteristics of children living in the city. We group administered the questionnaire in the classroom setting. All the schools were located in the city of Girona – a middle-size city according to Spanish standards, about 73.000 inhabitants. We obtained a sample of 968 students (13.2% of 12-olds, 22.5% of 13-olds, 26.7% of 14-olds, 23% of 15-olds and 14.6% of 16-olds). 478 are boys (49.4%) and 490 girls (50.6%).

Consistently with ethical guidelines for the conduct of research in Spain, first of all school directors and presidents of the parents association of each selected school were contacted to ask for permission. Next step was to contact teachers responsible for each class-room group and then a letter was addressed to each parent.

During the session, about an hour long, children's regular teacher and one or two researchers were present. Children were kindly asked for co-operation and were informed that data would be treated confidentially. And, of course, they had the right to refuse participating.

Measures

Overall and domain satisfaction with life

Seven items exploring satisfaction with specific domains were included in the questionnaire. Domains were: satisfaction with school performance, with learning, with time use, with amusing, with preparation for future, with the family, with friends. Additionally, an item on overall life satisfaction was also included. All these variables were measured through a five-point Likert scale, value 1 meaning "very dissatisfied" and 5 "very satisfied".

Values

One technique that has been used to explore children's aspirations is asking children to what extent they would like to be appreciated for some concrete values, when they get older. We have used this technique in previous research in order to identify different value structures between parents and children (Casas et al., 2003). For the present study we designed a closed set of items referred to aspirated values of children when they become 21 years old. Twelve values were studied: intelligence, technological skills, social skills, computers knowledge, profession value, family value, sensitivity, sympathy, money, power, knowledge of the world and own image. Variables regarding values were measured through a five-point Likert scale, value 1 meaning "not at all" and 5 "very much".

Perceived control

When we designed this exploratory research, we looked for a short scale, in order not to make a too long questionnaire. Therefore, we decided to use Pearly and Schooler's Mastery Scale (1978) as indicator of perceived control. This seven-item scale evaluates, according to the authors, potential life-strains that previous research had revealed to be commonly experienced in major social role areas, and the coping repertoires people employ in dealing with the strains they experience in these roles.

Behavioural intentions: Strategies to get information from the Internet

The option of planning or searching by chance on the Internet has been analysed through the answers to the following open-ended question: *to get information you look for on the Internet, do you think you have to plan your search carefully, or is it better to search by chance?* Most children using the Internet did answer using the expression "*to plan*", "*by chance*" or "*both*". Despite the possibility of giving a wider explanation, only very few gave a detailed one. Categorization was worked and tested by the members of the research team, obtaining more than 99% of coincidence. Answers were categorized in 5 groups: plan the search, random search, both are used, no answer (no Internet use) and non-valid answer. The analysis of this variable in this paper only includes the three first groups of answers (N = 605).

Statistical Analysis

According to the exploratory aim of this research, we use multivariate descriptive analysis techniques, chief among them principal component analysis (Pearson, 1901; for an introduction see for instance Dunteman, 1989). Varimax rotation was selected as specially suited to principal component analysis because it produces uncorrelated dimension scores and maximizes the interpretability of principal components subject to this restriction. According to the usual procedures, the selection of the number of dimensions was based on their interpretability and on the scree plot of percentages of explained variance. Principal components of different analyses were related by means of Pearson correlations. Principal components were related to categorical variables by means of ANOVA models. In these two latter cases, p-values are reported but must only be interpreted as a measure of strength of relationship, due to the non probabilistic character of the sample.

RESULTS

Principal Component Analysis of Satisfaction with Different Life Domains, and Correlation with Overall Satisfaction with Life

Principal Component Analysis with all variables in the questionnaire evaluating satisfaction with specific domains has been developed. A three-dimension structure explains the 70.79% of the total variance. Dimension I, which we have named *Enjoying time*

TABLE I

Results of the Principal Components Analysis of different life domains

Rotated Component Matrix

	Component		
	1	2	3
Satisfaction with school performance	4.254E-02	0.864	–1.820E-02
Satisfaction with learning	0.111	0.733	0.368
Satisfaction with time use	0.805	0.324	–8.184E-02
Satisfaction with amusing	0.793	3.653E-02	0.291
Satisfaction with preparation for future	0.425	0.588	0.241
Satisfaction with family	0.114	0.287	0.845
Satisfaction with friends	0.591	–3.899E-02	0.550

satisfaction is related to freedom of time use and includes satisfaction with time use, with amusing and with friends. Three items are outstanding components of Dimension II, that we have named *Learning related satisfaction*: satisfaction with school performance, satisfaction with learning and satisfaction with preparation for future. Lastly, Dimension III that we have named *Family satisfaction* is mainly loaded by the item satisfaction with family (see Table I).

When crossing these three dimensions with gender, only the relation with learning related satisfaction appears to be significant (t = 3.419; $p = 0.001$) in the sense that girls express more satisfaction than boys. The ANOVA test considering age shows significant relations with learning related satisfaction ($F_{4,925} = 9.177$; $p < 0.0005$) and family satisfaction ($F_{4,925} = 2.479$; $p = 0.043$). MDS (Minimum Difference Significance) post-hoc contrasts indicate that the youngest students in the sample show more learning related satisfaction than the oldest. Levels of family satisfaction are not so different when age is considered. However, between the most satisfied respondents (12 and 13-olds) and the least satisfied ones (15-olds), significant differences are observed.

In Table II the observed positive and significant correlation – not very high, though – between the three – satisfaction with life domains dimensions and satisfaction with life as a whole is shown.

TABLE II

Correlation of dimensions of domain satisfaction with overall satisfaction with life

Dimensions	Pearson	Significance
Enjoying time satisfaction	0.382	$p < 0.0005$
Learning related satisfaction	0.375	$p < 0.0005$
Family satisfaction	0.328	$p < 0.0005$

Principal Component Analysis of Values

Principal Component Analysis of the 12 items asking children about different values they would like to be appreciated in the future offers a good solution when classifying the variables into three groups. The total variance explained by the three-dimension structure is 56.75%. Money, power and image are mainly loaded in Dimension I, that we have named *Materialistic values.* Dimension II, that we named *Capacities and knowledge values*, is mainly loaded by intelligence, technical skills, computer knowledge, profession and knowledge of the world. Those values included in Dimension III, named *Interpersonal relationships values* are the following: social skills, family, sensitivity and sympathy (see Table III).

In accordance to expected gender stereotypes, boys express significantly higher emphasis in materialistic values dimension (t = 5.445; $p < 0.0005$) and capacities and knowledge values dimension (t = 4.900; $p < 0.0005$), whereas girls do in interpersonal relationships values dimension (t = 7.383; $p < 0.0005$). In contrast, when considering age differences, they are located in interpersonal relationships values dimension ($F_{4,911} = 2.848$; $p = 0.023$) in the sense that the youngest consider interpersonal relation values significantly less important for their future life than the oldest, with the 14-olds just in the middle by age and values.

Principal Component Analysis of the Perceived Control Scale

Two dimensions are extracted from the analysis considering the mastery psychometric scale, which explain the 53.77% of the

TABLE III

Results of the Principal Components Analysis of values

Rotated Component Matrix	Component		
	1	2	3
Intelligence value	–2.218E-03	0.705	0.275
Technological skills value	0.117	0.711	0.146
Social skills value	–4.240E-02	0.476	0.559
Computers knowledge value	0.242	0.709	–0.125
Profession value	0.238	0.515	0.333
Family value	0.247	0.133	0.576
Sensitivity value	1.461E-02	–1.339E-02	0.792
Sympathy value	1.812E-02	0.217	0.706
Money value	0.902	8.195E-02	8.696E-03
Power value	0.894	0.118	1.163E-02
Knowledge of the world value	0.393	0.451	0.198
Own image value	0.683	0.203	0.163

total variance. Those dimensions are Dimension I, named *External perceived control* and Dimension II, named *Internal perceived control*. We have not found any significant relation with gender, nor with age.

Correlation between Value Dimensions, Internal/External Perceived Control Dimensions and Satisfaction with Life as a Whole

Satisfaction with life as a whole is significantly correlated to value Dimensions II, *Capacities and knowledge values*, and III, *Interpersonal relationships values*, but not to Dimension I, *Materialistic values*. Correlations are positive and not very high (see Table IV).

The internal perceived control dimension is significantly and positively correlated with satisfaction with life as a whole. Interestingly, in the case of the external perceived control dimension, the relation observed is just the other way round (see Table V).

TABLE IV

Correlation of value dimensions with overall satisfaction with life

Dimensions	Pearson	Significance
Materialistic values	0,013	$p = 0.69$
Capacities and knowledge values	**0,154**	$\mathbf{p < 0.0005}$
Interpersonal relationships values	**0,098**	$\mathbf{p = 0.003}$

TABLE V

Correlation of internal/external perceived control dimensions with overall satisfaction with life

Dimensions	Pearson	Significance
External perceived control	**–0.289**	$\mathbf{p < 0.0005}$
Internal perceived control	**0.277**	$\mathbf{p < 0.0005}$

Correlation between Value Dimensions, Satisfaction Dimensions, and Perceived Control Dimensions

Relation between satisfaction dimensions – *enjoying life, learning related satisfaction, and family satisfaction* –; value dimensions – *materialistic values, capacities and knowledge values, and interpersonal relationships values* –; and perceived control dimensions – *external perceived control, and internal perceived control* – were examined. According Tables VI, VII and VIII, Pearson coefficients show significant and positive correlation between the following dimensions:

- enjoying time satisfaction and materialistic values,
- enjoying time satisfaction and capacities and knowledge values,
- enjoying time satisfaction and interpersonal relationships values,
- learning related satisfaction and capacities and knowledge values,
- external perceived control and materialistic values,
- internal perceived control and enjoying time satisfaction,

TABLE VI

Correlation between value dimensions and satisfaction dimensions

Satisfaction dimensions	Value dimensions		
	Materialistic values	Capacities and knowledge values	Interpersonal relationships values
Enjoying time satisfaction	**R = 0.082** **p = 0.015**	**R = 0.1** **p = 0.003**	**R = 0.139** **p < 0.0005**
Learning related satisfaction	**R = –0.078** **p = 0.02**	**R = 0.215** **p < 0.0005**	R = –0.055 p = 0.103
Family satisfaction	R = –0.024 p = 0.485	R = –0.03 p = 0.370	**R = –0.164** **p < 0.0005**

TABLE VII

Correlation between perceived control dimensions and satisfaction dimensions

Satisfaction dimensions	Perceived control dimensions	
	External perceived control	Internal perceived control
Enjoying time satisfaction	**R = –0.134** **p < 0.0005**	**R = 0.164** **p < 0.0005**
Learning related satisfaction	**R = –0.229** **p < 0.0005**	**R = 0.182** **p < 0.0005**
Family satisfaction	**R = –0.091** **p = 0.008**	**R = 0.143** **p < 0.0005**

- internal perceived control and learning related satisfaction,
- internal perceived control and family satisfaction, and
- internal perceived control and capacities and knowledge values.

Whilst the following variables present significant negative correlation:

TABLE VIII

Correlation between value dimensions and perceived control dimensions

Perceived control dimensions	Value dimensions		
	Materialistic values	Capacities and knowledge values	Interpersonal relationships values
External perceived control	**R = 0.078** **p = 0.023**	**R = –0.062** p = 0.07	R = 0.053 p = 0.122
Internal perceived control	R = –0.017 p = 0.623	**R = 0.167** **p < 0.0005**	**R = 0.171** **p < 0.0005**

- learning related satisfaction and materialistic values,
- family satisfaction and interpersonal relationships values,
- external perceived control and enjoying time satisfaction,
- external perceived control and learning related satisfaction,
- external perceived control and family satisfaction, and
- internal perceived control and interpersonal relationship values.

Relation between Satisfaction, Values and Strategies of Getting Information on the Internet

The original variable in our questionnaire evaluating satisfaction with life as whole was explored separately in relation to the options of planning, by chance searching, or both, on the Internet using the Kendall TAU-C test. A relationship between styles of getting information and satisfaction with life as a whole is found ($t_c = -0.072$; $p = 0.018$). Apart from showing the association between the variables mentioned, the negative sign indicates that the more satisfaction expressed by respondents, the more tendency to plan.

The ANOVA test between styles of getting information from Internet and the three identified satisfaction domains dimensions, show that significant differences are just found in relation to Dimension II, '*Learning related satisfaction*' ($F_{(2,583)} = 11.06$; $p < 0.0005$). Subjects in our sample who tend to rely on chance are significantly more dissatisfied with school, compared to the two other groups' respondents (those who tend to plan or to use indistinctly both styles).

No significant relation has been found when considering separately the original variables in our questionnaire evaluating different aspirated values of the adolescents in our study and searching strategies on the Internet. Consistently, the crossing between the three value dimensions and such strategies does not show any relationship either.

We have finally analysed the relationship between the external/internal perceived control dimensions above obtained and the option of planning or by chance searching information on the Internet. The ANOVA analysis reveals significant differences for the first dimension ($F_{(2,570)} = 5.554$; $p = 0.004$) and for the second ($F_{(2,570)} = 3.713$; $p = 0.025$). In both cases, the differences are located between those who prefer to plan and those who rely on chance. Those subjects who prefer to rely on chance show higher punctuation in external perceived control, whereas respondents in our sample, who prefer to plan, show higher internal perceived control.

DISCUSSION

Our results show once again that overall life satisfaction is related with satisfaction with different life domains, although correlations are rather low, indicating that life as a whole is not simply the sum of the life domains. In our sample, enjoying time satisfaction seems to contribute a little more to overall satisfaction with life than learning related satisfaction, and more than family satisfaction – these three dimensions being the most important ones we have identified.

A newer contribution appears when we analyse children's satisfaction with life as a whole in relation to children's personal aspirated values in the future. The more an adolescent in our sample considers non-materialistic values as very important, the more he or she seems to be satisfied with his or her life as a whole. However, when an adolescent aspirates to be highly valued for his/her materialistic achievements (money, power, and image) we cannot predict anything about his or her life satisfaction. Several tentative explanations are possible here. One is that individuals having high aspirations related to materialistic values may feel very far away from their goals when they are under 16, and for that reason their satisfaction with life as a whole should be related to other factors. An alternative explanation could be that individuals more highly satisfied with life are only seldom interested in materialistic values, whilst they are often interested in non-materialistic.

However, when we go into the detail of the concrete domain satisfaction dimensions in relation to each value dimension, we observe that enjoying time satisfaction correlates positively with all values. Whilst satisfaction with family only correlates with interpersonal relationships values, and satisfaction with learning related activities correlates with the other dimensions but not with interpersonal relationships values. In the studied period of the adolescence it seems possible to be satisfied enjoying time independently of own values. However, it seems that it is only possible to be very satisfied with family if the subject appreciates interpersonal relationships; and it seems it is difficult to appreciate interpersonal relationships if the subject only appreciates materialistic values or capacities and knowledge values.

On the other hand, and in this case also confirming previous research, adolescents higher in external perceived control appear to be less satisfied with life as a whole than those higher in internal perceived control. Individuals having internal perceived control are more likely to report they are satisfied with their overall life, and also with learning related aspects and with family, and are less likely to report high satisfaction with enjoying time.

Individuals with higher internal perceived control tend to aspirate to be valued for their capacities and knowledge, while those with higher external perceived control tend to aspirate to be valued for materialistic aspects. Another interesting result is that individuals higher in internal perceived control tend less to aspirate to be valued by interpersonal relationships values.

When we analyse intended strategies to action, the landscape that appears in front of us looks like a fish biting its tail: Children with external attribution (usually more unsatisfied with life) are more frequently using "by chance" strategies, that will probably lead them more often to unsatisfactory fulfilment of their aspirations.

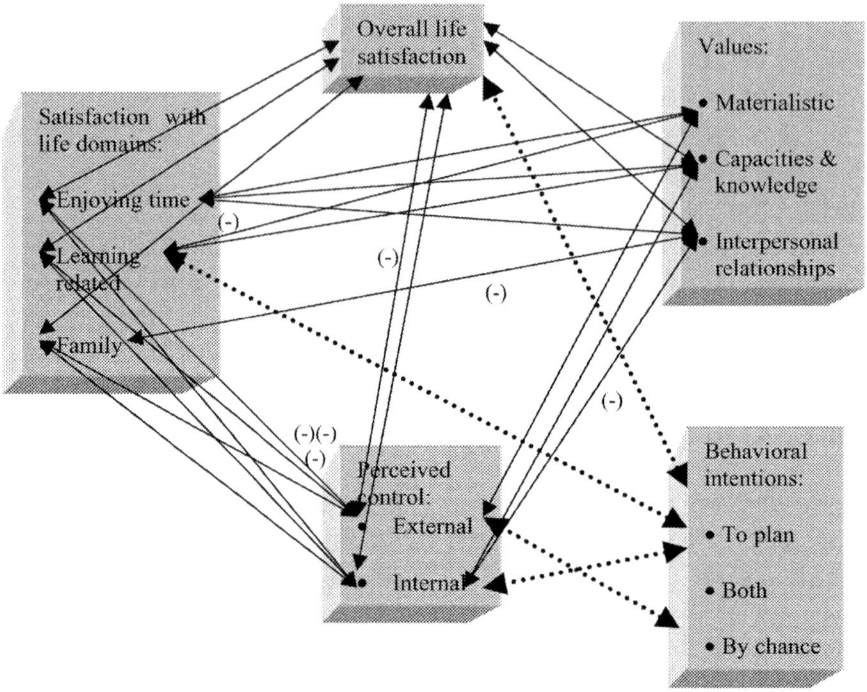

Figure 2. Pearson significant correlation (continuous-line arrows) among identified dimensions of the constructs explored in this study and Kendall TAU-C or ANOVA significant relations identified (dot-line arrows).

Children more often intending to use the strategy of planning their action tend to be more satisfied with their learning related activities, with their preparation for the future, with their family and with their overall life.

However, no relation appears between intended strategies to fulfil the own goals and values. Such results are surprising, and seem to be in disagreement with the quoted literature on that topic. One possible interpretation is that for children 12 to 16 years old strategies used to reach intended goals have nothing to do with own values, suggesting that general aspirations and concrete aspirations may function independently, although mediated by subjective well-being and perceived control.

All these correlation identified are reflected in Figure 2, that gives us some clarification about the complex interrelations among the constructs we have included in Figure 1. Our hypothesis stating that values have some kind of relationship with satisfaction with life

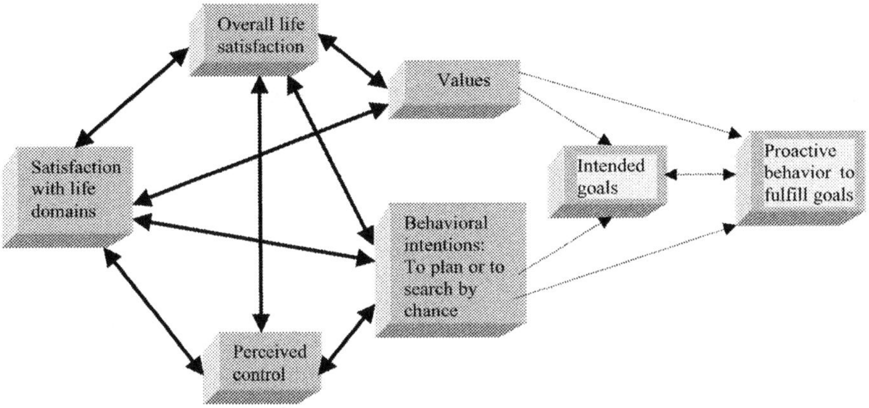

Figure 3. Relationships found among the constructs explored in this study (continuous-line arrows) and hypothetical related constructs (dot-line arrows) to be explored in the future.

domains and satisfaction with life as a whole is clearly supported. Overall life satisfaction shows a relation with behavioural intentions about to plan or not to plan action to fulfil intended goals.

Last but not least, perceived control is confirmed as a key construct to understand the relations between well-being of adolescents and their behavioural intentions about to plan or not to plan the fulfilment of their intended goals.

Main limitations of the current study include demographic features of the sample, the difficulties linked to the answers of adolescents to a unique open-ended item and the fact that only self-reported data are available. In relation to the sample, participants have been recruited from only one area, thus making the results difficult to be generalised to the behaviour of, at least, Spanish adolescents. Second, different formulations and a broader set of items should be explored in the future. Lastly, the possible existence of a method bias due to self-reported data is another aspect to be aware of.

Several directions for future research stem from the limitations above mentioned. First of all, it is desirable in the near future to extend this study to other samples, and even to adolescents of different cultural backgrounds. Second, the use of discussion groups and in-depth interviews with adolescents should be employed in order to have different types of data to be compared, and thus, allow us to deepen in our knowledge of the complex relationships among the variables studied in this article. In this sense, the analysis of the relationships among the constructs explored in this study with the real proactive behaviours to fulfil own goals in the case of the adolescent population, is still to be done (see Figure 3). Structural Equation Models should be used with this purpose.

REFERENCES

Campbell, A., P.E. Converse and W.L. Rodgers: 1976, The Quality of American Life: Perceptions, Evaluations and Satisfactions (Russell Sage Foundation, New York).

Casas, F., C. Alsinet and M. Rosich: 1999, 'Análisis del bienestar psicológico de los niños y niñas. Las escalas de satisfacción vital y las escalas de afecto positivo y negativo', V Congreso Estatal de Intervención Social 3, pp. 2071–2081.

Casas, F., C. Figuer and M. González and G. Coenders: 2003, 'Satisfaction with life domains and salient values for future among children and their parents in 5 different countries', 5th Conference of the International Society for Quality-Of-Life Studies.

Casas, F., M. Rosich and C. Alsinet: 2001, 'El bienestar psicológico de los preadolescentes', Anuario de Psicología 31(2), pp. 73–86.

Casas, F., C. Alsinet, M. Rosich, E.S. Huebner and J.E. Laughlin: 2000, 'Cross-cultural investigation of the Multidimensional Life Satisfaction Scale with Spanish adolescents', Third Conference of the International Society for Quality of Life Studies. Girona, 20–22 July 2000.

Dunteman, G.H.: 1989, Principal Components Analysis (Sage, Thousand Oaks, CA).

Friedman, S.L., E.K. Scholnick and R.R. Cocking: 1987, 'Reflections on reflection: What planning is and how it develops', in S.L. Friedman, E.K. Scholnick and R.R. Cocking (eds.), Blueprints for Thinking: The Role of Planning in Cognitive Development (Cambridge University Press, Cambridge, UK), pp. 515–534.

Friedman, S.L. and E.K. Scholnick: 1987, 'Setting the stage: An integrative framework for understanding research on planning', in S.L. Friedman and E.K. Scholnick (eds.), The Developmental Psychology of Planning: Why, How, and When Do We Plan? (Lawrence Erlbaum, Mahwah, NJ), pp. 3–22.

Garzón, A. and J. Garcés: 1989, 'Hacia una conceptualización del valor', in A. Rodríguez and J. Seoane (eds.), Creencias, actitudes y valores (Alhambra, Madrid).

Hart, R.A.: 1992, Children's Participation. From Tokenism to Citizenship. Innocenti Essays, 4. Florence. I.C.D.C. UNICEF.

Huebner, E.S.: 1991, 'Correlates of life satisfaction in children', School Psychology Quaterly 6, pp. 103–111.

Huebner, E.S.: 1994, 'Preliminary development and validation of a multidimensional life satisfaction scale for children', Psychological Assessment 6, pp. 149–158.

Huebner, E.S. and T. Dew: 1993, 'Validity of the perceived life satisfaction scale', School Psychology International 14, pp. 355–360.

Kreitler, S. and H. Kreitler: 1987, 'Concepts and processes of planning: Their motivational and cognitive antecedents', in S.L. Friedman, E.K. Scholnick and R.R. Cocking (eds.), Blueprints for Thinking: The Role of Planning in Cognitive Development (Cambridge University Press, Cambridge, UK), pp. 110–178.

Martín, S., J.M. Martínez, J.S. López, M.J. Martín and J.M. Martín: 1998, 'Comportamientos de riesgo: violencia, prácticas sexuales de riesgo y consumo de drogas ilegales' (Emtinema, Madrid).

Nurmi, J.E.: 1991, 'How do adolescents see their future? A review of the development of future orientation and planning', Developmental Review 11, pp. 1–59.

Nurmi, J.E.: 1993, 'Adolescent development in an aged-graded context: The role of personal beliefs, goals and strategies in the tackling of developmental tasks and standards', International Journal of Behavioral Development 16, pp. 169–189.

Pearly, L. and C. Schooler: 1978, 'The structure of coping', Journal of Health and Social Behaviour 19, pp. 2–21.

Pearson, K.: 1901, 'On lines and planes of closest fit to a system of points in space', Philosophical Magazine, Series 6, pp. 559–572.

Pinillos, J.L.: 1982, 'El cambio de los sistemas de valores en las sociedades desarrolladas y en las sociedades en desarrollo', Reunión Internacional sobre Psicología de los Valores. Policopied.

Rokeach, M.: 1973, The Nature of Human Values (Free Press, New York).

Skinner, E.A.: 1997, 'Planning and perceived control', in S.L. Friedman and E.K. Scholnick (eds.), The Developmental Psychology of Planning: Why, How, and When Do We Plan? (Lawrence Erlbaum, Mahwah, NJ), pp. 263–284.

Skinner, E.A. and J.P. Connell: 1986, 'Control understanding: Suggestions for a developmental framework', in M.M. Baltes and P.B. Baltes (eds.), The Psychology of Control and Aging (Lawrence Erlbaum, Hillsdale, NJ), pp. 35–69.

Institut de Recerca sobre Qualitat de Vida (IRQV)
Universitat de Girona
Pl. S. Domènec, 9
17071-Girona
Spain
E-mail: ferran.casas@udg.es

RICH GILMAN, SUSAN R. EASTERBROOKS and MICHELE FREY

A PRELIMINARY STUDY OF MULTIDIMENSIONAL LIFE SATISFACTION AMONG DEAF/HARD OF HEARING YOUTH ACROSS ENVIRONMENTAL SETTINGS

ABSTRACT. A key aspect of life quality is life satisfaction. Interest in this construct has increased among children and adolescents over the past decade given the differential mental health and educational outcomes associated with life satisfaction reports. Nevertheless, most research has used general samples of students, with very little understood of how youth with disabilities view the quality of their lives. Further, many students with disabilities live and/or are educated in totally segregated residential schools or segregated day school programs. It is thus unclear how life satisfaction reports may differ with respect to these environmental settings. Using the *Multidimensional Students' Life Satisfaction Scale*, global satisfaction, as well as satisfaction ratings across a number of life domains was compared among Deaf/Hard-of-Hearing (D/HH) youth living in residential settings and D/HH youth attending day school programs. These reports were also compared with a group of hearing peers. Results revealed that the inter-domain correlations, regression coefficients, and satisfaction mean scores varied between the disability and non-disability groups, and with respect to environmental setting. Implications of these findings conclude the paper.

Quality of life is a universal construct that encompasses many factors (Felcer, 1997). For years, research investigating quality of life among groups has focused on objective indicators, such as income level, gender, and crime statistics, among others. However, sole focus on objective indicators only accounts for a portion of the variance (Diener et al., 1999), suggesting that quality of life is largely regulated by internal mechanisms, rather than by objective experiences (Bearsley and Cummings, 1999). Increasing research has thus focused on subjective aspects in order to gather unique information that is not captured by objective indicators alone (Diener and Suh, 1997; Veenhoven, 1996). Expressed satisfaction with life (i.e., cognitive appraisal of one's life based on an individual's own selected standards: Campbell et al., 1976) is one such

Social Indicators Research **66:** 143–164, 2004.

aspect that is considered to be a key indicator of life quality (Diener and Diener, 1995; Felcer, 1997).

A number of explanations highlight the importance of life satisfaction when assessing quality of life. First, life satisfaction encompasses but also transcends the immediate effects of life events (Heady and Wearing, 1992) and mood states (Seidlitz et al., 1997), adding unique variance not accounted for by solely assessing affect (i.e., positive and negative emotions). Second, life satisfaction is less ephemeral than the affective state (Diener and Diener, 1995) and is more stable over time (Diener, 2000). Third, life satisfaction is not simply an outcome of other psychological states, but influences important psychosocial systems as well. For example, in a longitudinal study with adults, Lewinsohn et al. (1991) reported that low life satisfaction predicted the onset of depression two to three years earlier. Moum (in Diener, 2000) also reported that low life satisfaction predicted suicide over the following five years. Further, changes in life satisfaction have also been related to health status (Veenhoven, 1988) and occupational functioning (Marks and Fleming, 1999). Finally, interventions specifically designed to enhance life satisfaction have resulted in positive outcomes in response to stress (Frederick, 2001) and poor physical health (Seaman, 1989). These findings collectively suggest that life satisfaction appraisals not only result from an interplay of personal and environmental conditions, but also in turn influence subsequent internal and environmental experiences (Diener et al., 1999).

Although still in its infancy, research investigating life satisfaction among children and adolescents has also increased. Research using this age group is important considering the presence of relevant harmful behaviors (drug use, youth violence, etc.) and negative stressors (peer conflicts, family conflicts) that may contribute to substantial declines in life quality for many youth (Arnett, 1999; Collins, 1991). As support for the utility of life satisfaction research, a number of negative and positive outcomes have been associated with youth satisfaction reports including depression (Lewinsohn et al., 1991), anxiety (Gilman et al., 2000), health and risk behaviors such as alcohol/illicit drug use (Zullig et al., 2001), violent behavior (Valois et al., 2001), and social stress (Neto, 1993) (see Gilman and Huebner, in press, for an overall review of life satisfaction research). Given these findings, assessing students' life satisfaction across a variety of relevant life domains may allow researchers and clinicians to design strategies that promote the well-being of youth who remain dissatisfied with their lives (Baker et al. 1997; Huebner et al., 2000).

To date, studies investigating satisfaction have largely utilized general samples of school-age students. Although such studies are important in their own right, various authors contend that enhanced life quality should be considered primary goal of *every* youth, including those with disabilities (Brown, 1999; Green and Reid, 1999; Griffin and Huebner, 2000). A common goal among parents (and society) is for their child to achieve their hopes and dreams, to be healthy, to choose good friends, and to lead productive lives as adults (Helm, 2000). However, for youth with disabilities, a number of barriers may be placed before them that render these goals especially difficult to attain. For example, through continued interactions and relationships with parents, peers, teachers, and others, youth with disabilities face their 'differentness' on a daily basis and may experience constrained autonomy that potentially compromises their life quality (Szymanski, 2000). Although research investigating the quality of life (including life satisfaction) among students with disabilities remains in its nascent stage, there is some indication that life satisfaction reports among students with disabilities differ across some life domains in comparison to their non-disabled peers. For example, Griffin and Huebner (2000) found that middle school students diagnosed with severe emotional disturbance reported significantly lower satisfaction with their friends than normally achieving students (see also Adelman et al., 1989). Similar findings have also been reported among students diagnosed with mild mental disabilities (Brantley et al., in press).

In light of these recent findings, claims regarding the utility of life satisfaction reports must be continually evaluated with respect to a wide array of disabilities. The disability group of interest in this study was youths who were deaf or hard-of-hearing (D/HH), a term that encompasses a broad range of hearing loss and one that is assigned regardless of communication preference (i.e., sign language) or cultural affiliation (Isrealite et al., 2002). Although a heterogeneous group, the unifying theme among the D/HH population is substantial impairment in auditory functioning that makes understanding oral communication difficult or impossible to attain. As a result, a number of stressors are experienced that may interfere with normal psychological development, including optimal parent-child (Ita, 1999) and peer-child relationships (Cartledge et al., 1991; Stinson and Liu, 1999), school difficulties (Isrealite et al., 2002), and interpersonal distress and low self-worth (Dessell, 1994; Obrzut et al., 1999; Zieziulz and Harris, 1998). The etiological mechanisms that cause hearing loss may be of less clinical importance than communication difficulties and deficits in social relationships that are commonly associated with the disorder (Cartledge et al., 1991; Munoz-Baell and Ruiz, 2000). It is these difficulties that may serve to increase the risk of psychological distress among D/HH youths while concomitantly diminishing their life quality (Brubaker and Szakowski, 2000).

As has been noted by others (Diener, 1996; Veenhoven, 1996), life satisfaction is not a stochastic phenomenon but fluctuates in response to environmental contexts (see Bearsley and Cummins, 1999; Marshall et al., 1996). In the case of D/HH youth, one factor that may influence life satisfaction is the environmental context in which the youth is educated. If an environment does not foster a sense of belongingness or support positive interactions with peers, teachers, and parents, it is likely that the D/HH youth will view his/her condition as particularly stigmatizing (Warrick, 1994). This circumstance may contribute to low life satisfaction across a number of domains. Conversely, D/HH youth who are largely in supportive environments may view their condition as less of a "handicap", and thus positive self-identity is not compromised (Israelite et al., 2002; Leigh et al., 1998; Munoz-Baell and Ruiz, 2000). This supportive environment may, in turn, lead to enhanced life satisfaction.

Discussions abound advocating for the inclusion of D/HH children in public school settings (e.g., Cambra, 2002; Stinson and Liu, 1999) and, in fact, approximately 72% of youth with hearing loss are educated in regular education environments (Gallaudet Research Institute, 2002). Nevertheless, placement in more restrictive settings continues and has elicited comments from proponents and critics alike regarding its psychosocial benefits. On the one hand, proponents argue that segregated environments facilitate easier, greater, and more meaningful communication between children, peers, educators, and parents (Cartledge et al., 1991), and foster more positive social interactions and a greater sense of belongingness (Stinson, Whitmire and Kluwin, 1996). On the other hand, critics of segregated settings argue that placement reinforces the view that D/HH is stigmatizing. Further, critics contend that placement in segregated settings severely restricts opportunities for youth to acquire social behaviors that would be acceptable to the dominant hearing culture, thus contributing to lower life quality across many areas of their lives including relationships with parents, peers, and school experiences (see Bat-Chava, 2000; Cartledge et al., 1991; Mertens, 1989).

Although some studies have investigated the relationship between life quality and educational placement among non D/HH youth and D/HH youth in public schools (see Kluwin et al., 2002), no research has specifically assessed the construct of life satisfaction, nor has any study compared multidimensional life satisfaction reports between D/HH youth educated and/or living in different environments (i.e., day schools and segregated residential schools) with their non-D/HH peers. To address this void in the literature, the present study first compared multidimensional life satisfaction reports among a group of D/HH students with a general group of hearing youths in order to determine if life satisfaction varied with respect to hearing status. In addition, multidimensional life satisfaction reports were compared between D/HH students in residential schools (where there is little contact with the home environment) and in segregated day school settings (where the students maintain routine family involvement). These ratings were again compared to the non-D/HH group.

METHOD

Participants

A total of 159 students served as participants in the study. The total sample ranged between 8 and 18 years of age ($M = 13.04$, $SD = 2.94$) and was comprised of 82 males and 77 females, of which 134 were Caucasian, 8 were African-American, and 17 were labeled as 'other' (i.e., Hispanic-American, Asian-American, Native-American). The mean grade level of the sample was 6.86 ($SD = 2.74$). The majority of youth (65%) were from socioeconomic backgrounds whose income levels ranged between $20000 and $80000. Seventy-one students comprised the non-D/HH sample, with the mean age being 11.14 ($SD = 2.00$). There were 37 males and 34 females, of which 65 were Caucasian, 2 African-American, and 4 labeled as 'Other'. The D/HH day school group was selected from one segregated day school in a large metropolitan area in the Southeast. A total of 23 students from this group participated in the study. The mean age was 13.22 ($SD = 2.51$). There were 12 males and 11 females, of which 13 were Caucasian, 2 African-Americans, and 7 classified as 'other'. The D/HH residential group was obtained from one state residential setting in the Midwest ($N = 25$) and one state residential setting in the Northeast ($N = 40$). There were a total of 33 males and 32 females. The mean age was 15.06 ($SD = 2.51$). Fifty-five students were Caucasian, 4 students were African-American, and 6 students were classified as 'Other'. Independent sample T-tests between the two residential settings across variables of interest did not significantly differ. Thus, the residential settings were combined in order to preserve statistical power.

Procedure

Only students who were either granted permission from the institution (i.e., the state residential school from the Northeast) or returned a signed parental consent and student assent form participated in the study. In all settings, the administration of the life satisfaction instrument was conducted in a small classroom setting under the supervision of the third author and/or trained assistants. For the non-D/HH group, in order to minimize any problems due to reading difficulties, the directions were first read aloud prior to the students completing the instrument. For both D/HH groups, a videotape of a person signing each item of the instrument was presented as an option to the students. The items were signed in American Sign Language (ASL) and transliterated in Conceptually Accurate Signed English (CASE). When needed, the students followed along with the videotape, and answered the relevant items. For all groups, students were instructed to think about their lives over the past several weeks when rating each item. The students were allowed to complete the instrument at their own pace, with the third author or trained assistants remaining present throughout to answer any questions the students had.

Instrument

The Multidimensional Students' Life Satisfaction Scale (MSLSS: Huebner, 1994) is a 47-item self-report instrument that assesses satisfaction across five specific life domains (family, friends, school, living environment, self) as well as a global domain (i.e., questions not pertaining to a specific life domain). All questions on the MSLSS are responded to on a six-point Likert response format (1 = strongly disagree, 2 = moderately disagree, 3 = mildly disagree, 4 = mildly agree, 5 = moderately agree, 6 = strongly agree). Scoring of each domain is obtained by summing the relevant items and then dividing by the number of items comprising each domain. Negatively worded items are reverse-ordered so that a higher score is indicative of higher levels of satisfaction. Studies of the MSLSS have consistently demonstrated acceptable psychometric properties across grades 3–12, including stability coefficients ranging from 0.77 to 0.86 for each domain (Huebner and Gilman, in press; Gilman and Huebner, 2000), strong evidence of construct validity as determined by both confirmatory (e.g., Gilman et al., 2000; Huebner et al., 1998) and exploratory factor analyses (Dew, 1996), and strong evidence for convergent validity (Huebner et al., 1998). The reading level of the MSLSS has been estimated to be at the third-grade level (Huebner, 1994). In order to reflect the living situation of the D/HH children in residential settings and to facilitate ease in interpretation, select items on the MSLSS Friends, School, and Living Environment scales were slightly modified. For example, "I wish I had different friends" was modified to become "I wish I had different friends at [name of residential school]".

Given the reservations concerning the interpretation of items on psychological instruments for D/HH youth (Obrzut et al., 1999; Vernon and Miller, 2001), the internal consistency of the MSLSS was first analyzed for all three groups. For the non-D/HH group, coefficient alphas ranged from 0.76 (Family) to 0.84 (Global), which were similar to results obtained from other studies (e.g., Gilman and Huebner, 2000) and met the 0.70 criteria considered appropriate for research purposes (Salvia and Ysseldyke, 1988). With the exception of the Global domain (α = 0.55), the internal consistencies of the MSLSS domains among the D/HH day school group were appropriate for research purposes, with coefficient alphas ranging from 0.70 (Living Environment) to 0.77 (School, Family). Nevertheless, the low internal consistency of the Global domain suggests some caution in interpreting global satisfaction for this group. For the D/HH residential setting group, internal consistency among the MSLSS domains estimates ranged between 0.70 (School, Self) to 0.77 (Family), with the exception of the Friends domain (α = 0.55). Caution is suggested when interpreting this particular domain for this group.

RESULTS

Independent samples T tests were first analyzed between the D/HH group (as a whole) and the non-D/HH group in order to determine if multidimensional satisfaction reports differed with respect to hearing status. Because some students omitted answering one or two items on the MSLSS, listwise deletions resulted in different sample sizes across domains. Levene's Test for Equality of Variance was significant for the School, Family, and Living Environment domains and thus significance testing for these particular domains was computed after taking into account the unequal group sizes. In order to control for Type I errors, the alpha was Bonferonni corrected to 0.008 (0.05/6). Table I reports the mean domain satisfaction scores for the two groups as well as the results of the independent T-tests. With the exception of the Self and School satisfaction domains, differences between the two groups across MSLSS domains were significant. Further, and regardless of statistical significance, the non-D/HH group reported higher mean scores on most MSLSS domains than the combined D/HH group.

Pearson correlations were then analyzed to determine the amount of shared variance with respect to the MSLSS domain for non-D/HH students and D/HH students placed in their respective educational setting (see Table II). The pattern of correlations for the non-D/HH group very closely matched what has been reported in previous studies (e.g., Gilman et al., 2000; Gilman and Ashby, 2002). Inter-

TABLE I

Means and standard deviations (in parentheses) of the MSLSS domain scores for the combined D/HH group and non-D/HH group

Satisfaction domains	N	df	Mean (SD)*	T-Test	sig.
Global					
D/HH	86	155	3.74 (0.88)		
Non-D/HH	71		4.54 (1.08)	5.18	0.000
Friends					
D/HH	84	151	4.43 (0.80)		
Non-D/HH	69		5.31 (0.76)	6.94	0.000
Self					
D/HH	82	149	4.78 (0.79)		
Non-D/HH	69		5.05 (0.70)	2.24	0.027
School					
D/HH	86	155	4.42 (1.18)		
Non-D/HH	71		4.40 (1.06)	–0.06	0.950
Living environment					
D/HH	79	140	3.84 (1.37)		
Non-D/HH	69		4.65 (0.97)	4.22	0.000
Family					
D/HH	83	146	4.61 (1.05)		
Non-D/HH	71		5.74 (0.73)	3.56	0.000

MSLSS = Multidimensional Students' Life Satisfaction Scale. D/HH = Deaf/Hard of Hearing.
*MSLSS scoring is based on a 6-point Likert rating scale where 1 = strongly disagree, 2 = moderately disagree, 3 = mildly disagree, 4 = mildly agree, 5 = moderately agree, 6 = strongly agree.

domain correlations were also moderate at best for both D/HH groups, suggesting that the domains were discriminate (but not orthogonal) and were in keeping with the underlying theoretical structure of life satisfaction (Huebner, 1994). The largest correlation for the non-D/HH group was the relationship between global and family satisfaction ($r = 0.67$). While this particular relationship was also significant among the D/HH day school group ($r = 0.53$),

TABLE II

Bivariate correlations of the MSLSS domains across group

	Global	Friends	Self	Family	Living env.	School
Non-D/HH						
Global	—					
Friends	0.52**	—				
Self	0.61**	0.52**	—			
Family	0.67**	0.37**	0.57**	—		
Living env.	0.38**	0.46**	0.39**	0.43**	—	
School	0.46**	0.24*	0.49**	0.46**	0.47**	—
D/HH day school						
Global	—					
Friends	0.24	—				
Self	0.29	0.51*	—			
Family	0.53**	0.60**	0.51*	—		
Living env.	0.47**	0.51*	0.29	0.47*	—	
School	0.20	0.71**	0.34	0.50*	0.34	—
D/HH residential setting						
Global	—					
Friends	0.26*	—				
Self	0.39*	0.54**	—			
Family	0.12	0.43**	0.52**	—		
Living env.	0.30	0.07	0.13	0.06	—	
School	0.14	0.09	0.12	0.23	0.71**	—

*$p < 0.05$; **$p < 0.01$.

the relationship between school and friendship satisfaction yielded the highest correlation ($r = 0.71$). For the D/HH residential group, several non-significant correlations were obtained and the pattern of coefficients was dissimilar than either the non-D/HH group or the D/HH day school group. For example, neither the moderate relationship between global and family satisfaction for the non-D/HH group was found for the D/HH residential group ($r = 0.12$). Further, unlike the D/HH day school group, the relationship between school and friendship satisfaction was not significant for the D/HH residential group ($r = 0.09$). The largest magnitude of shared variance for the D/HH residential group was noted between satisfaction with school and living environment ($r = 0.71$). In general, these particular findings demonstrate that the relationship between life satisfaction domains vary not only with respect to hearing status but also across environmental setting.

A standard multiple regression was next conducted, with each D/HH group dummy coded and compared with the non-D/HH group (who served as the reference group in the regression equation). Separate analyses were conducted for each MSLSS domain, and the results are presented in Table III. Although the standardized coefficients are reported in the table for the sake of completeness, their interpretation is often less meaningful in dummy coding procedures. Thus, unstandardized coefficients are considered more useful to interpret (Cohen and Cohen, 1983). Significant R differences were noted on the Global domain, $F(2, 156) = 13.41$, $p < 0.001$, and the Friends, $F(2, 152) = 25.46$, $p < 0.001$, Family, $F(2, 153) = 5.98$, $p < 0.001$, and the Living Environment domains, $F(2, 156) = 10.29$, $p < 0.001$. Of the significant findings, and in order of magnitude, 25% (24% adjusted) of the variance was predicted by the D/HH groups on the Friends domain, followed by the Global and Living Environment domains. Further, the significant differences were largely based on responses from the D/HH residential group than from the D/HH day school group. For example, among the D/HH residential group, the coefficients for the Global, Friends, and Living Environment domains were different in magnitude by almost a full point above that provided by the intercept alone (i.e., the mean domain scores of the non D/HH group). The unstandardized coefficients from the D/HH day school group contributed less additional information over that provided by the intercept. Further, mean scores from the D/HH residential group contributed unique variance that was higher in magnitude across the significant domains in comparison to the D/HH day school group ($sr^2 = 0.77$ and $sr^2 = 0.03$ for Global satisfaction; $sr^2 = 0.50$ and $sr^2 = 0.12$ for Friends; $sr^2 = 0.26$ and $sr^2 = 0.02$ for Family, and $sr^2 = 0.35$ and $sr^2 = 0.15$ for Living Environment satisfaction for the D/HH residential and D/HH day school group respectively).

TABLE III

Multiple regression analysis of MSLSS domains by disability group

MSLSS domain	B	β	F	sig.	R^2	R^2_{adj}
Global						
Non D/HH	3.71*					
D/HH day school	0.08	0.03	13.41	0.001	0.15	0.14
D/HH residential	0.83	0.40				
Friends						
Non D/HH	4.35					
D/HH day school	0.29	0.12	25.46	0.001	0.25	0.24
D/HH residential	0.95	0.54				
Self						
Non D/HH	4.79					
D/HH day school	–0.03	–0.02	2.51	>0.05	0.03	0.02
D/HH residential	0.26	0.17				
School						
Non D/HH	4.39					
D/HH day school	0.09	0.03	0.06	>0.05	0.01	0.01
D/HH residential	0.02	0.01				
Family						
Non D/HH	4.59					
D/HH day school	0.05	0.02	5.98	0.001	0.07	0.06
D/HH residential	0.53	0.23				
Living environment						
Non D/HH	3.68					
D/HH day school	0.54	0.16	10.29	0.001	0.12	0.11
D/HH residential	0.97	0.39				

*Coefficients reported for the non-D/HH group refers to the constant (intercept) in the regression equation.

Finally, a between-subjects multivariate analysis of covariance compared the MSLSS domains for each D/HH group and the non-D/HH group. Adjustment was made for the covariates of age, race, and gender. Table IV reports the raw means and standard deviations of the MSLSS domains across group and setting. The results yielded a significant main effect, Pillai's Trace = 0.29, $F(6, 130) = 3.71, p <$

TABLE IV

Means and standard deviations (in parentheses) of the MSLSS domain mean scores across group and setting

	D/HH (day school)	D/HH (residential)	Non-D/HH	F	sig.	ES
Global	3.80 (0.74)[a]	3.71 (0.93)[a]	4.54 (1.08)[b]	13.41	0.001	0.15
Friends	4.64 (0.91)[a]	4.34 (0.34)[a]	5.31 (0.76)[b]	25.45	0.001	0.25
Self	4.75 (0.86)	4.79 (0.76)	5.05 (0.70)	2.51	>0.05	0.03
School	4.49 (0.99)	4.39 (1.25)	4.40 (1.06)	0.06	>0.05	0.01
Living env.	4.21 (0.91)[a]	3.68 (1.52)[b]	4.65 (0.97)[a]	10.29	0.001	0.12
Family	4.65 (0.97)[a]	4.59 (1.08)[a]	5.13 (0.73)[b]	5.98	0.004	0.07

Rows not sharing the same superscript significantly differ at the 0.01 level. N (D/HH day school) = 23; N (D/HH residential) = 63; N (non-D/HH group) = 71.

0.000, with the multivariate effect size considered small ($\eta^2 = 0.16$). None of the covariates were significantly related to the combined dependent variables, revealing that scores on all MLSS domains were invariant with respect to demographic variables.

Follow-up univariate tests after adjustment for covariates (and Bonferroni corrected to 0.004 in order to limit Type I errors) revealed significant main effects on the Global domain, $F(2, 140) = 13.41$, $p < 0.001$, and the Friends, $F(2, 140) = 25.45$, $p < 0.001$, Living Environment, $F(2, 140) = 10.29$, $p < 0.001$, and Family satisfaction domains, $F(2, 140) = 5.98$, $p < 0.004$. The highest effect size was obtained on the Friends domain ($\eta^2 = 0.25$). Similar to the findings when the D/HH groups were combined, equivalent self and school satisfaction ratings were reported regardless of group and environmental setting. However, with the exception of school satisfaction, non-D/HH children reported higher satisfaction scores across all MSLSS domains in comparison to both D/HH groups, and their global satisfaction and satisfaction with their friends and family was significantly higher than either D/HH group. Further, the mean living environment satisfaction score was significantly different between the non-D/HH group and the D/HH residential group, but was not significantly different between the non-D/HH group and the D/HH day school group. Although both D/HH groups reported equivalent mean global, friends, and family satisfaction scores, the D/HH group reported significantly higher living environment satisfaction than the D/HH residential group.

DISCUSSION

A number of findings reported herein are considered noteworthy. To begin, the analysis of the descriptive data revealed that D/HH youth, as a collective group, reported lower life satisfaction scores across most MSLSS domains than their hearing peers. These mean score differences were statistically significant with respect to global satisfaction, as well as satisfaction with family, friends, and living environment. The differences in global satisfaction are viewed with particular importance given that this domain is rather sensitive to life circumstances (Bearsley and Cummins, 1999; Gilman and Barry, in press). Considering that the mean global score for the D/HH group was the lowest among the MSLSS domains, the present results suggest that a number of these youth were experiencing less than optimal overall life quality, insofar as comparison to their hearing peers are concerned. Further, the importance of family and friendships on the positive development of children and adolescents has been well documented (Franco and Levitt, 1998; Masten, 2001). Such relationships are considered particularly important among D/HH youth, where communication difficulties may be a source of frustration and contentious relationships between D/HH youth and important individuals in their lives (Powers and Saskiewicz, 1998; Mertens, 1989). Although recent research has reported no differences in quality of parenting between children with hearing disorders and their hearing peers, many of these studies only solicited responses from parents (e.g., Brubaker and Szakowski, 2000; Powers and Saskiewicz, 1998), thus omitting valuable information of family quality from the youths' perspective. Based on the current self-reports, the results from this study revealed that qualitative differences in family satisfaction existed between D/HH and their hearing peers, with higher satisfaction noted among the non-D/HH group. Further, the difference in mean scores between the two groups on friendship satisfaction was the largest among all mean scores, indicating that fundamental differences existed in the quality of peer relations and social support. Considering that this was the first study to investigate life satisfaction among a sample of D/HH youth, future studies are needed to establish the generalizeablility of these findings. Specific aspects of parenting and/or friendship quality are also needed to understand factors that are necessary for positive appraisals regarding these specific domains.

In addition to the differences in multidimensional life satisfaction that were reported between disability and non-disability group, significant differences were also noted after separating each disability group into their primary educational setting. In many respects, life satisfaction reports appeared to yield more sensitivity for the D/HH residential group than for the D/HH day school group. Specifically, an examination of the correlation matrix revealed that the pattern and magnitude of correlations for the non-D/HH group and the D/HH day school group were roughly similar. As one example, the relationship between global and family satisfaction for both groups was similar and paralleled findings reported elsewhere (Gilman at al., 2000). However, the pattern and magnitude of the correlations were much different among the D/HH residential group. For example, the relationship between family and global satisfaction was minimal, as were other correlations that yielded significance for the other two groups. What was highly significant for the D/HH residential group (but less so for the other two groups) was the relationship between living environment and school (capturing almost 50% of the total variance between the two variables). This particular finding illustrates the relative strength of school and living environment satisfaction among D/HH youths in total segregated environments, in comparison to D/HH youths in less segregated environments or their hearing peers. It may be the case that the relatively limited amount of time that D/HH youths living in residential settings leads them to view their school, staff, and peers as their "surrogate family".

Further, the results of the regression analysis yielded unstandardized coefficients and unique predictors that were different and more pronounced among the D/HH residential group than among the D/HH day school group (in comparison to the intercept of the non-D/HH group). Specifically, the coefficients for the D/HH residential group were almost a full point different from the intercept on global satisfaction, and satisfaction with friends and living environment. Most of the coefficients among the D/HH day school group contributed negligible additional information over that provided by the intercept. Further, the magnitude of the unique variance on global satisfaction and satisfaction with friends, family, and living environment was greater among the D/HH residential group than their peers in day school settings.

Although the nature and correlates of multidimensional life satisfaction appeared to be different between the two disability groups, a comparison of the MSLSS domains revealed that the only significant mean score difference was found on the Living Environment domain, with the D/HH residential group reporting significantly lower satisfaction than the D/HH day school group. Satisfaction with living environment was not significantly different between the D/HH day school group and the non-D/HH group. Although the effect size of this difference is considered to be statistically small, the qualitative labeling of the mean living environment satisfaction score for the non-disabled group and the less segregated D/HH day school group was equivalent to the response option of "moderately agree", while the mean score for the D/HH residential group was roughly equivalent to "mildly agree". Previous studies using the MSLSS have classified groups of students solely based on their collective mean scores (e.g., students from the "mildly agree" group versus the "moderately agree" group), and these groups have been shown to vary on psychoeducational outcomes (e.g., Gilman, 2001; Huebner et al., 2000). Thus, while the differences in mean scores may be statistically small, the practical significance of the differences awaits further research.

Although differences in living environment satisfaction scores between D/HH groups provided some support for the aforementioned shortcomings inherent to placement in totally segregated environments (e.g., Cartledge et al., 1991), the contention that life quality is compromised across various domains (e.g., friends, family) as a result of such placement was not supported. Indeed, equivalent school and self satisfaction mean scores were reported regardless of disability status and/or environmental placement, indicating that the youth collectively reported relatively high acceptance of their academic environment and personal characteristics. Further, there were no differences in global satisfaction and satisfaction with friends and family between the D/HH groups (although mean scores in these domains were significantly lower than the non-DHH group). Until further research is conducted, it can be maintained that D/HH youth in totally segregated settings view their overall satisfaction and satisfaction across many life domains as being no different than their D/HH peers in less segregated settings. Nevertheless, that the D/HH residential group reported significantly lower living environment satisfaction warrants further investigation of the potential reasons for these lower collective mean scores (e.g., quality of caregiving, qualitative analysis of residential settings, degree of acculteration into the deaf culture).

Some limitations of the study must be noted. First, interpretation of findings related to life satisfaction and living environment must be tempered the fact that this study is based on data collected on one occasion from a cross-section of students. How life satisfaction reports may have changed as a function of time spent in placement was not investigated. This variable is important to consider in future studies given preliminary evidence to suggest that multidimensional life satisfaction fluctuates in response to time spent in residential settings. For example, Gilman and Barry (in press) reported that children diagnosed with Oppositional Defiant Disorder reported significantly lower satisfaction across a number of life domains when first entering a residential treatment setting than three months post-admission. Although life satisfaction in general displays a moderate degree of stability (Diener et al., 1999), future research should incorporate longitudinal designs in order to be more sensitive to potential changes in life satisfaction reports among D/HH students in segregated environments. Relatedly, although the MSLSS domain scores were no different across the residential school settings, thus permitting greater confidence in the generalizeability of the findings for residential students, only one day school setting was used in the study. Future research is needed that incorporates additional day schools. Finally, the relatively small sample size of the clinical groups precluded matching of age, race, and/or gender with the non-D/HH group, and more sophisticated statistical procedures (e.g., confirmatory factor analysis) that would permit greater psychometric confidence in using the MSLSS for D/HH youth could not be conducted. Although the coefficient alphas of most MSLSS domains were similar to previous studies, the relatively lower internal consistency of the Global domain (D/HH day school group) and the Friends domain (D/HH residential school group) suggest caution in interpreting these findings. Given these limitations, this study should be interpreted as a preliminary attempt to assess life satisfaction among youth with a Dead/Hard of Hearing disability.

REFERENCES

Adelman, H.S., L. Taylor and P. Nelson: 1989, 'Minors' dissatisfaction with their life circumstances', Child Psychiatry and Human Development 20, pp. 135–147.

Arnett, J.J.: 1999, 'Adolescent storm and stress revisited', American Psychologist 54, pp. 371–386.

Baker, J.A., T. Terry, R. Bridger and A. Winsor: 1997, 'Schools as caring communities: A relational approach to school reform', School Psychology Review 26, pp. 586–602.

Bat-Chave, Y.: 2000, 'Diversity of deaf identities', American Annals of the Deaf 145, pp. 420–428.

Bearsley, C. and R.A. Cummins: 1999, 'No place called home: Life quality and purpose of homeless youths', Journal of Social Distress and the Homeless 8, pp. 207–226.

Bender, T.A.: 1997, 'Assessment of subjective well-being during childhood and adolescence', in G. Phye (ed.), Handbook of Classroom Assessment: Learning, Achievement, and Adjustment (Academic Press, San Diego, CA), pp. 199–225.

Brantley, A., E.S. Huebner and R.J. Nagle: in press, 'Multidimensional life satisfaction reports of adolescents with mild mental disabilities', Mental Retardation.

Brown, I.: 1999, 'Embracing quality of life in times of spending restrain', Journal of Intellectual and Developmental Disability 24, pp. 299–309.

Brubaker, R.G. and A. Szakowski: 2000, 'Parenting practices and behavior problems among deaf children', Child and Family Behavior Therapy 22, pp. 13–28.

Cambra, C.: 2002, 'Acceptance of deaf students by hearing students in regular classrooms', American Annals of the Deaf 147, pp. 38–43.

Campbell, A., P. Converse and W. Rodgers: 1976, The Quality of American Life (Russell Sage Foundation, New York).

Cartledge, G., P.V. Paul, D. Jackson and L.L. Cochran: 1991, 'Teachers' perceptions of the social skills of adolescents with hearing impairment in residential and public school settings', Remedial and Special Education 12, pp. 34–39.

Cohen, J. and P. Cohen: 1983, Applied Multiple Regression/Correlation Analysis for the Behavioral Sciences, 2nd ed. (Lawrence Erlbaum, Hillsdale, NJ).

Collins, J.K.: 1991, 'Research into adolescence: A forgotten era', Australian Psychologist 26, pp. 1–9.

Cowen, E.: 1994, 'The enhancement of psychological wellness: Challenges and opportunities', American Journal of Community Psychology 22, pp. 149–179.

Dew, T.: 1996, The preliminary development and validation of a multidimensional life satisfaction scale for adolescence, Unpublished doctoral dissertation, University of South Carolina, Columbia, SC.

Diener, E.: 1996, 'Traits can be powerful, but they are not enough: Lessons from subjective well-being', Journal of Research in Personality 30, pp. 389–399.

Diener, E.: 2000, 'Subjective well-being: The science of happiness and a proposal for a national index', American Psychologist 55, pp. 34–43.

Diener, E., and M. Diener: 1995, 'Cross-cultural correlates of life satisfaction and self-esteem', Journal of Personality and Social Psychology 68, pp. 653–663.

Diener E. and E.M. Suh: 1997, 'Measuring quality of life: Economic, social, and subjective indictors', Social Indicators Research 40, pp. 189–216.

Diener, E., Suh, E.M., Lucas, R.E., and Smith, H.L.: 1999, 'Subjective well-being: Three decades of progress', Psychological Bulletin 125, pp. 276–302.

Felcer, D.: 1997, 'Defining and applying the concept of quality of life', Journal of Intellectual Disability Research 41, pp. 126–135.

Franco, N. and M.I. Levitt: 1998, 'The social ecology of middle childhood: Family support, friendship quality, and self-esteem', Family Relations, 47, pp. 315–321.

Frederick, B.L.: 2001, 'The role of positive emotions in positive psychology: The broaden-and-build theory of positive emotions', American Psychologist 56, pp. 218–226.

Gallaudet Research Institute: 2002, Regional and National Summary Report of Data From 2000–2001: Annual Survey of Deaf and Hard of Hearing Children and Youth (Gallaudet University, Washington, DC).

Gilman, R.: 2000, 'The relationship between life satisfaction, social interest, and frequency of extracurricular activities among adolescent students', Journal of Youth and Adolescence 30, pp. 749–767.

Gilman, R. and J.S. Ashby: 2002, 'A study of perfectionism and multidimensional life satisfaction among adolescents', manuscript submitted for publication.

Gilman, R. and J. Barry: in press, 'Multidimensional life satisfaction and social desirability among adolescents in a residential treatment setting: Changes across time', Residential Treatment for Children and Youth.

Gilman, R. and M.L. Handwerk: 2001, 'Changes in life satisfaction as a function of stay in a residential setting', Residential Treatment for Children and Youth 18, pp. 47–65.

Gilman, R. and E.S. Huebner: in press, 'Life satisfaction among children and adolescents: A review of the research', School Psychology Quarterly.

Gilman, R. and E.S. Huebner: 1999, 'Review of life satisfaction measures for adolescents', Behaviour Change 17, pp. 178–195.

Gilman, R., E.S. Huebner and J.E. Laughlin: 2000, 'A first study of the Multidimensional Students' Life Satisfaction Scale with adolescents', Social Indicators Research 52, pp. 135–160.

Green, C.W. and D.H. Reid: 1999, 'A behavioral approach to identifying sources of happiness and unhappiness among individuals with profound mental disabilities', Behavior Modification 23, pp. 280–294.

Greenspoon, P.J. and D.H. Saklofske: 1997, 'Validity and reliability of the Multidimensional Students' Life Satisfaction Scale with Canadian children', Journal of Psychoeducational Assessment 15, pp. 138–155.

Griffin, M.D. and E.S. Huebner: 2000, 'Multidimensional life satisfaction reports of middle school students with serious emotional disturbance', Journal of Psychoeducational Assessment 18, pp. 111–124.

Heady, B. and A. Wearing: 1992, Understanding Happiness: A Theory of Subjective Well-being (Longman Cheshire: Melbourne, Victoria, Australia).

Helm, D.T.: 2000, 'The measurement of happiness', American Journal of Mental Retardation 105, pp. 326–335.

Huebner, E.S.: 1994, 'Preliminary development and validation of a multidimensional life satisfaction scale for children', Psychological Assessment 6, pp. 149–158.

Huebner, E.S., W. Drane and R.F. Valois: 2000, 'Levels and demographic correlates of adolescent life satisfaction reports', School Psychology International 21, pp. 281–292.

Huebner, E.S., J.E. Laughlin, C. Ash and R. Gilman: 1998, 'Further validation of the Multidimensional Students' Life Satisfaction Scale', Journal of Psychoeducational Assessment 16, pp. 118–134.

Israelite, N., J. Ower and G. Goldstein: 2002, 'Hard-of-hearing adolescents and identity construction: Influences of school experiences, peers, and teachers', Journal of Deaf Studies and Deaf Education 7, pp. 134–148.

Ita, C.M.: 1999, 'The psychological development of children who are deaf or hard of hearing: A critical review', Volta Review 101, pp. 165–182.

Kluwin, T.N., M.S. Stinson and G.M. Colarossi: 2002, 'Social processes and outcomes of in-school contact between deaf and hearing peers', Journal of Deaf Studies and Deaf Education 7, pp. 200–213.

Larson, R.W.: 2000, 'Toward a psychology of positive youth development', American Psychologist 55, pp. 170–183.

Lazarus, R.S.: 1991, Emotion and Adaptation (Oxford University Press, New York).

Leigh, I.W., A.L. Marcus, P.K. Dobosh and T.E. Allen: 1998, 'Deaf/hearing cultural identity paradigms: Modification of the Deaf Identity Development Scale', Journal of Deaf Studies and Deaf Education 3, pp. 329–338.

Lewinsohn, P., J. Redner and J. Seeley: 1991, The relationship between life satisfaction and psychosocial variables: New perspectives', in F. Strack, M. Argyle and N. Schwartz (eds.), Subjective Well-Being (Plenum Press, New York), pp. 193–212.

Marks, G.N. and N. Fleming: 1999, 'Influences and consequences of well-being among Australian young people: 1980–1995', Social Indicators Research 46, pp. 301–323.

Marshall, G.N., M.A. Burnam, P. Koegel, G. Sullivan and B. Benjamin: 1996, 'Objective life circumstance and life satisfaction: Results from the course of homelessness study', Journal of Health and Human Behavior 37, pp. 44–58.

Masten, A.S.: 2001, 'Ordinary magic: Resilience processes in development', American Psychologist 56, pp. 227–238.

Mertens, D.M.: 1989, 'Social experiences of hearing-impaired high school youth', American Annals of the Deaf 134, pp. 15–19.

Munoz-Baell, I.M. and M.T. Ruiz: 2000, 'Empowering the deaf: Let the deaf be deaf', Journal of Epidemiology and Community Health 54, pp. 40–44.

Musselman, C., A. Mootilal and S. MacKay: 1996, 'The social adjustment of deaf adolescents in segregated, partially integrated, and mainstreamed settings', Journal of Deaf Studies and Deaf Education 1, pp. 52–63.

Neto, F.: 1993, 'The Satisfaction with Life Scale: Psychometrics properties in an adolescent sample', Journal of Youth and Adolescence 22, pp. 125–134.

Obrzut, J.E., G.J. Maddock and C.P. Lee: 1999, 'Determinants of self-concept in deaf and hard of hearing children', Journal of Development and Physical Disabilities 11, pp. 237–251.

Powers, G.W. and J.A. Saskiewicz: 1998, 'A comparison study of educational involvement of hearing parents of deaf and hearing children of elementary school age', American Annals of the Deaf 143, pp. 35–39.

Salvia, J. and J.E. Ysseldyke: 1988, Assessment in Special and Remedial Education, 3rd ed. (Houghton Mifflin, Boston, MA).

Seidlitz, L., R.S. Wyer and E. Diener: 1997, 'Cognitive correlates of subjective well-being: The processing of valenced life events by happy and unhappy persons', Journal of Research in Personality 31, pp. 240–256.

Selkever, D.S.: 2000, 'Activity status, life satisfaction, and perceived productivity for young adults with developmental disabilities', Journal of Rehabilitation 66, pp. 4–14.

Stinson, M.S. and Y. Liu: 1999, 'Participation of deaf and hard-of-hearing students in classes with hearing students', Journal of Deaf Studies and Deaf Education 4, pp. 191–202.

Stinson, M.S., K. Whitmire and T.N. Kluwin: 1996, 'Self-perceptions of social relationships in hearing-impaired adolescents', Journal of Educational Psychology 88, pp. 132–143.

Szymanski, L.S.: 2000, 'Happiness as a treatment goal', American Journal of Mental Retardation 105, pp. 352–362.

Valois, R.F., K.J. Zullig, E.S. Huebner and J.W. Drane: 2001, 'Relationship between life satisfaction and violent behaviors among adolescents', American Journal of Health Behavior 25, pp. 353–366.

Veenhoven, R.: 1996, 'Developments in satisfaction research', Social Indicators Research 37, pp. 1–46.

Veenhoven, R.: 1988, 'The utility of happiness', Social Indicators Research 20, pp. 333–354.

Vernon, M. and K. Miller: 2001, 'Interpreting in mental health settings: Issues and concerns', American Annals of the Deaf 146, pp. 429–433.

Zullig, K.J., R.F. Valois, E.S. Huebner, J.E. Oeltmann and J.W. Drane: in press, 'Relationship between perceived life satisfaction and adolescent substance abuse', Journal of Adolescent Health.

Department of Educational and Counseling Psychology
245 Dickey Hall, College of Education Building
University of Kentucky
Lexington, KY 40506
USA
E-mail: gilman@uky.edu

SHANNON M. SULDO and E. SCOTT HUEBNER

THE ROLE OF LIFE SATISFACTION IN THE RELATIONSHIP BETWEEN AUTHORITATIVE PARENTING DIMENSIONS AND ADOLESCENT PROBLEM BEHAVIOR

ABSTRACT. Research examining environmental factors associated with adolescents' life satisfaction (LS) has revealed that familial variables (e.g., parent-child conflict, family structure) are crucial correlates. The purpose of the current study was to identify particular dimensions of authoritative parenting (strictness-supervision, social support/involvement, and psychological autonomy granting) that are related to LS during early, middle, and late adolescence, as well as to explore the hypothesis that LS serves as a mediator between authoritative parenting and adolescent internalizing and externalizing behavior. A sample of 1201 middle and high school students completed self-report measures assessing these constructs. Results indicated statistically significant relationships between each authoritative parenting dimension and adolescent LS. Although all three parenting dimensions were positively related to LS, perceived parental social support emerged as the strongest correlate. Important developmental differences were revealed, including the finding that the association between parenting behaviors and adolescents' LS changed as children aged. Last, LS fully mediated the relationship between social support and adolescent problem behavior and partially mediated relationships between the remaining authoritative parenting dimensions (i.e., strictness-supervision, psychological autonomy granting) and maladaptive adolescent behavior.

After years of focusing on pathology, the field of psychology appears ready for change. For instance, the first issue of the *American Psychologist* in the 21st century was dedicated to "happiness, excellence, and optimal human functioning". This publication set the tone for psychology research in the new millennium by stressing the importance of positive indicators of functioning, as opposed to equating well-being with an absence of deviant behavior.

One research domain especially pertinent to positive functioning involves the study of subjective well-being (SWB). Three related, yet distinguishable, constructs (positive affect, negative affect, and life satisfaction) have been traditionally assumed to comprise SWB (Diener, 2000). Positive affect refers to pleasant feelings and moods,

Social Indicators Research **66:** 165–195, 2004.

while negative affect describes emotions that are bothersome and/or disagreeable. Specific definitions of life satisfaction (LS) vary, but Diener (1994) asserts that global LS reflects a cognitive judgment of one's satisfaction with life as a whole. The distinctness of positive affect, negative affect and LS has been confirmed, partially by research that has demonstrated that factors, such as self-concept and life events, differentially influence these three SWB variables (e.g., McCullough, Huebner and Laughlin, 2000).

Justification for studying life satisfaction is initially provided through face validity – that is, who can fault psychologists for examining factors that enhance people's overall contentedness? While psychologists have produced an abundance of information on LS in adults, this avenue of research has been substantially less traveled with respect to children and adolescents. Although children have always been worthy beneficiaries of research on LS, recent tragedies involving childhood expressions of anger at school serve to hasten a focus on improving the well-being of youth. The importance of identifying manipulable contextual factors (e.g., parents' behaviors, peer behavior) that might predict the occurrence of such tragedies is thus particularly salient. This research examines one contextual influence, the impact of the parent-child system, on adolescent LS and the potential mediating role of LS in occurrences of externalizing and internalizing behaviors.

Preliminary studies with children and youth focused on identifying demographic, personality, and environmental correlates of life satisfaction. Collectively, demographic factors (e.g., gender, SES, age, race) are relatively weak predictors of children's LS (Gilman and Huebner, 1997; Huebner, 1991a; Sam, 1998; Wilson, Henry and Peterson, 1997). Several personality variables including self-esteem, locus of control, and extraversion are significantly associated with children's LS (Heaven, 1989; Huebner, 1991a; McCullough, Huebner and Laughlin, 2000; Wong and Csikszentmihalyi, 1991). Environmental variables significantly related to LS in children and adolescents include neighborhood (Homel and Burns, 1989), culture (Sam, 1998), stressful life events (McCullough et al., 2000), special education status (Adelman et al., 1989; Huebner and Alderman, 1993) and, in particular, several familial factors.

Important Role of Family Functioning in Adolescents' Life Satisfaction

Despite the emphasis on peer relationships, physical appearance, and schooling in adolescence, research with this age group indicates that attainment of LS is more strongly associated with positive relationships with *parents*, a finding that holds across multiple societies. For example, Dew and Huebner's (1994) research with American adolescents found perceived quality of relationships with parents was the strongest predictor of their LS, proving more important than perceived physical appearance, general self-concept, and peer relations. Quality of parent-child relations is also paramount in determining Chinese adolescents' LS (Leung and Leung, 1992; Shek, 1997a). For instance, research with youth in Hong Kong found that the quality of the parent-child relationship was a stronger predictor of LS than the quality of relationships between adolescents and their same-age friends or school experiences (Leung and Zhang, 2000; Man, 1991). In addition, Sastre and Ferriere's (2000) research on family structure and subjective well-being in French adolescents found that the average LS score for children living at home with their parents is twenty percent higher than the mean satisfaction level of their agemates who have been removed from their homes. In sum, it appears that family relationships exert great influence on adolescents' LS in several cultures.

Specific family-related factors associated with adolescent LS include family structure, parent-child conflict, social support, and authoritative parenting. Preliminary research suggested that children from married or continuously single-parent (i.e., never married or divorced) families have superior well-being (as measured by a single mother-report item concerning her child's global welfare) than children living in divorced or stepfamilies (Demo and Acock, 1996). On the other hand, Grossman and Rowat (1995) found that perceived poor parental relationships, rather than family status, predicted low LS in adolescents from both married and divorced homes. Thus, witnessing a loveless parental relationship appears to be more detrimental to children's well-being than does divorce.

Concerning parent-child conflict, Demo and Acock (1996) found that the strongest predictor of adolescent global well-being was mother-adolescent disagreement, which exerted a greater influence than family structure (i.e., married, divorced) or parental relations. Research including assessments of paternal relationships found that while discord between children and both mothers and fathers was negatively associated with adolescents' LS, father-child conflict had a slightly stronger impact on LS than mother-child conflict (Shek, 1997b).

Early investigations of the association between parent-child relations and adolescent well-being focused on parental support. Specifically, Burke and Weir (1979) examined the role of parental responses to adolescents' requests for assistance. Parents who offered concrete support, giving explicit advice or suggestions, had children with higher levels of self-reported LS, while parents who were domineering or critical of their child's problems negatively impacted their LS. Furthermore, LS was elevated in adolescents satisfied with the informal help/support offered by their parents (Burke and Weir, 1978). Recent research with pregnant teenagers revealed that young women who both received support from, and provided support to, their parents reported significantly higher LS than pregnant teenagers who did not perceive this bidirectional parental support (Stevenson et al., 1999). Interestingly, this study also found that varying levels of social support to and from *friends* did not affect the LS of the pregnant teenagers. Focusing on parental support, Young and colleagues (1995) examined the differential impact of three types of social support on adolescent well-being and found that intrinsic support (i.e., the child's perception that the parent loves, appreciates, and cares about him or her) correlates more strongly with adolescents' LS than extrinsic support (i.e., monetary support and physical contact) or closeness (i.e., the child's perceived emotional bond to the parent).

Prior to the twenty-first century, the only direct examination of the influence of specific authoritative parenting behaviors on adolescent well-being operationalized "well-being" as low scores on a depression inventory (McFarlane et al., 1995). This preliminary study revealed that adolescent reports of parental care were negatively correlated with depression scores, whereas parental overprotection was positively related to depressive symptoms. In 2000, Petito and Cummins published the first study to link authoritative parenting to a positive measure of adolescent well-being, i.e., overall subjective quality of life (SQOL). Children who perceived authoritative parenting, defined as a relationship in which decision making is a joint process between parent and child but with parents' reserving the final judgment, had significantly higher SQOL scores than children who perceived their parents to be unengaged (e.g., adolescents responsible for decision making). While this study provides important information, it did not examine the potentially differential relationships between adolescents' LS and separate dimensions of authoritative parenting.

To summarize, examining such environmental variables as residence, culture, stressful life events, situational factors, and family results in numerous significant correlates of children's LS. Moreover, parent-child relationships and a general authoritative style of parenting have been found to be particularly strong predictors. Given the multidimensionality of authoritative parenting (Baumrind, 1991; Gray and Steinberg, 1999; Steinberg et al., 1989), additional research is needed to delineate the relative importance of the respective dimensions of authoritative parenting. Thus, current theories from developmental psychology regarding specific dimensions of authoritative parenting should be incorporated into research of children's LS.

Authoritative Parenting

Early theories asserted that two dimensions of parenting behaviors, *responsiveness* and *demandingness*, account for much of children's growth during adolescence (Baumrind, 1991). Responsiveness measures parents' degree of sensitivity, supportiveness, and involvement, whereas demandingness refers to the degree to which parents hold high expectations for their adolescents' behavior while monitoring their activities. Baumrind's research indicated that an *authoritative* parenting style, which is high in both characteristics, is most likely to produce adolescents who are socially competent, self-reliant and responsible. Conversely, parents who are neither responsive nor demanding are labeled *neglectful*, and have adolescents with increased behavior problems and decreased attention to school. *Authoritarian* parenting (high demandingness, low responsiveness) results in adolescents who have few problems with behavior or school, but are less self-reliant and self-confident. Finally, parents who are responsive but undemanding, referred to as *indulgent*, generally raise children who are socially adept and peer-oriented, yet display behavior problems and a decreased interest in school.

Building on the work of Baumrind, Steinberg and his associates (1992, 1999) assert that parenting styles involve *three* dimensions. The first, *acceptance-involvement*, corresponds to Baumrind's responsiveness factor, in that it refers to the extent to which adolescents feel their parents are loving, responsive, and involved. The remaining two factors, *strictness-supervision* and *psychological autonomy granting*, contain components that Baumrind combined in her demandingness category. Specifically, strictness-supervision refers to *behavioral* control through monitoring and limit setting, while psychological autonomy granting involves encouraging adolescents' individuality and emotional autonomy by *reducing psychological* control. This conceptualization has proven theoretically important, as types of parental control yield different effects on adolescent outcomes, namely externalizing and internalizing behaviors. Authoritative parenting, which consists of high levels of acceptance-involvement, strictness-supervision, and psychological autonomy granting, leads to desirable outcomes like school success (i.e., academic improvement, heightened school engagement, academic self-competence, grade point average) (Gray and Steinberg, 1999; Steinberg et al., 1992). Further research is certainly warranted to elucidate which dimensions of authoritative parenting are most strongly related to LS in children and adolescents, as well as to determine whether LS mediates the influence of authoritative parenting on established outcome variables, such as internalizing and externalizing problems (Steinberg et al., 1991).

Objectives of the Present Study

The purpose of the current research was threefold. First, we desired to elucidate the relationships between specific dimensions of authoritative parenting and adolescents' LS. In this study, three dimensions (acceptance-involvement, strictness-supervision, and psychological autonomy granting) described by previous researchers (e.g., Baumrind, 1991; Schaefer, 1965; Gray and Steinberg, 1999) were used to explore authoritative parenting.

Acceptance-involvement/ In the current investigation, social support was selected as an indicator of parental responsiveness/involvement for several reasons. First, support is the only parenting behavior related to authoritative parenting that has been previously investigated with regard to adolescent LS. Thus, results from this study will augment an existing body of research (e.g., Burke and Weir, 1979; Liebkind and Jasinskaja-Lathi, 2000; Zimmerman et al., 1995). Additionally, in line with the goals of this study (i.e., delineate *specific* parenting behaviors predictive of LS), we aimed to identify particular types of support that may relate to adolescent LS. Social support is a multidimensional construct that refers to interpersonal relationships that provide companionship, assistance, attachment, and protection from stressful life events. Researchers have identified four main dimensions of support: emotional, informational, instrumental, and social companionship (Wills et al., 1996a). Indeed, prior research has found differential relationships between subtypes of support and LS (Stevenson et al., 1999; Young et al., 1995).

Strictness-supervision. Parental strictness-supervision refers to the extent to which parents monitor, supervise, and are aware of their adolescents' activities and whereabouts. The amount of parental supervision during adolescence strongly affects a child's behavior, with decreased rates related to increased delinquency (Gray and Steinberg, 1999; Patterson and Stouthamer-Loeber, 1984). Comparable studies relating strictness-supervision to youths' LS are absent.

Psychological autonomy granting. Psychological autonomy granting involves parental encouragement of adolescents' individuality through reducing psychological control. Successful promotion of psychological autonomy is associated with decreased adolescent internalizing problems, and increased adolescent self-reliance and self-esteem (Gray and Steinberg, 1999). While the relationship between autonomy granting and LS among minors is unknown, research with young adults found that parental psychological control was only significantly related to LS when the effect of parental acceptance was not controlled for (Seibel and Johnson, 2001).

The aforementioned study by Seibel and Johnson (2001) examined LS and authoritative parenting in a sample of college students and found that retrospective accounts of perceived parental acceptance were more predictive of young adults' current LS than other dimensions of authoritative parenting, namely psychological autonomy and limit setting. In light of findings in developmental psychology (i.e., significant relationships between each dimension of authoritative parenting and a variety of mental health outcomes in *adolescents*), we hypothesized that social support, strictness-supervision, and psychological autonomy granting would all provide sizeable, unique contributions to youths' LS.

A second goal of the current study was to examine the prospect of LS as a mediating variable between parents' behavior and adolescents' internalizing and externalizing behavior. A growing body of research has examined the correlates of children's LS, generally under the assumption that a variety of subjective personal and environmental variables influence one's LS. Likewise, longitudinal studies have chosen to study LS as an outcome variable, affected by such factors as personal goals and family environment (Shek, 1999; Stein and Newcomb, 1999). A separate body of research has explored the impact of environmental influences, particularly family, on children's behavior. To cite an instance, Lamborn and her colleagues (1991) determined the differential impact of parenting styles on adolescents' involvement in school misconduct, drug use, and delinquency.

It is conceivable that these two lines of research may be closely related, with LS serving as a mediating variable between environmental factors (e.g., authoritative parenting) and adolescents' behavior. A mediator is defined as "the generative mechanism through which the focal independent variable is able to influence the dependent variable of interest ..." (Baron and Kenny, 1986: p. 1173). Life satisfaction, which Diener (1994) asserts is a cognitive appraisal of one's overall contentment, may be one psychological means through which family relationships affect children's behavior. In other words, it is plausible that the manner in which parents relate to their offspring directly influences their adolescents' LS, which in turn affects adolescent behavior.

Recent empirical research has supported the notion that adolescents have the mental capacity to incorporate events from their environments into their global feelings and attitudes towards their selves, which, in turn, influence their activities. For example,

Brendgen, Vitaro, and Bukowski (1998) found that in young adolescents experiencing peer rejection, "the relation between perceived closeness with parents and friends' delinquent behavior was mediated by self-esteem" (p. 259). Thus, this study demonstrated that early adolescents have the cognitive capacity to internalize their parental interactions in an assessment of their self image which, in turn, impacted their choice of peers with whom to affiliate. Research has also established self-esteem as a cognitive variable through which social/environmental experiences (i.e., social support, stressful life events, parent-child conflict) influence adolescents' behavior problems and suicidal thoughts (DuBois et al., 1994; Shagle and Barber, 1995). Such studies support the role of cognitive mediators in the relationship between adolescents' environments and behaviors. Life satisfaction, a global assessment of one's life experiences, is another plausible mediator worthy of investigation.

Third, this study aimed to explore the role of adolescent development in the relationship between parenting and LS. To date, all investigations of the relationship between LS and parenting have neglected to examine potential developmental differences. Although a solitary term, 'adolescence', is commonly used to refer to the period between ages 11–19, a time when youth are contending with and achieving autonomy, this range includes prepubescent children and mature young adults. In response to the awareness that younger adolescents are more influenced by the physical changes of puberty and changing relationships with their family and peers, whereas older adolescents are more concerned with solidifying their own identity, modern researchers have advocated dividing this developmental period into segments such as early, mid, and late (Cobb, 1998). Due to the heterogeneity of this developmental period, any study that purports to generalize to 'adolescents' should attempt to include children from the entire age range in its sample. This is especially pertinent in family research; younger adolescents struggle to separate from their parents, while older adolescents are ready to respect and appreciate their parents as people (Smollar and Youniss, 1989). Consequently, particular parenting dimensions (e.g., strictness-supervision, social support) are likely to vary in their impact on adolescents of different ages. Accordingly, this study examined the differential impact of familial relationships on LS in early, middle, and late adolescence. We hypothesized that the influence of authoritative parenting dimensions would change as a function of the adolescents' age.

METHOD

Participants

Complete datasets were collected from 1201 students, ages 11 to 19 (*M* = 14.6; *SD* = 2.1), enrolled in grades 6 (15%), 7 (15%), 8 (13%), 9 (16%), 10 (16%), 11 (12%), and 12 (13%) in three middle schools and two high schools within a large public school system in South Carolina, USA. Following statistical detection of multivariate outliers, data from thirteen participants were excluded from this study. Thus, the final sample retained for all subsequent data analyses included 1188 adolescents. The subsample of early adolescents (26%) was comprised of 314 students ages 11 and 12. The middle adolescent subsample (43%) contained 510 students ages 13 to 15, and 364 students ages 16 to 19 comprised the late adolescent subsample (31%).

Letters describing the study and requesting permission for participation were sent to parents of all students enrolled (*N* = 4140) in the participating schools. The rate of students returning completed parent permission forms (*N* = 1344) varied from 30% to 34% by school, a proportion typical in studies that have employed this same consent procedure with children. Students with parental consent were given a student assent form that reviewed the study's purpose and the voluntary nature of participation, as well as stated that participating students would receive candy, a chance to win a $50 cash giveaway, and/or a free pizza. Most students (*N* = 1258) elected to participate and were present on data collection dates. Note that the sampling method employed in the current study does not yield a random sample and, therefore, p-values reported in subsequent text should be interpreted with caution; priority may be given to the size of estimates and semipartial correlation coefficients.

Consistent with the demographics of this rural community, most participants were African American (58%); the remaining were Caucasian (34%), Hispanic (2%), Asian (2%), Native American

(1%) or mixed-race (3%). The gender distribution was 64% female. Almost half of the participants resided with both biological parents (49%); the remaining lived with their mother only (24%), their mother and stepfather (15%), their father and stepmother (3%), their father only (3%), or other adults such as a member of their extended family (6%). As an estimate of socioeconomic status, 58% of the sample qualified for school lunch at free or reduced rate (low SES), while the remainder (42%) qualified for paid lunches (average and above-average SES).

Procedures

Students were administered each measure discussed below in groups of 20–100, with the size of the group depending upon the availability of sufficient space and adult assistance to promote full understanding of instructions and candid and confidential completion of the measures. The sequence of the measures was counterbalanced. Participants completed a brief demographic questionnaire concerning their gender, age, grade, race, family structure and SES (SES was assessed by a single item asking whether or not the student received a free or reduced-cost lunch). The first author was present at all administration sessions to insure the accurate distribution and confidential completion and collection of all measures.

Measures

Students' Life Satisfaction Scale (SLSS) (Huebner, 1991b). The SLSS consists of seven items assessing global LS. Students were instructed to respond to each item using a 6-point response format, on which responses ranged from include 1 = "strongly disagree" to 6 = "strongly agree". Items 3 and 4 are reverse scored, such that high scores on the SLSS represent high LS. Finally, all item responses are averaged in order to yield a mean LS score between 1 and 6.

The SLSS is a reliable and valid measure with students in elementary, middle, and high school (for a review, see Bender, 1997). Coefficient alphas have been reported to be above .80 for 4th through 12th graders (Gilman and Huebner, 1997; Huebner, 1991b). Coefficient alpha in the current study was 0.83. Huebner (1991b) reported high stability coefficients for early adolescents: a two-week test-retest coefficient of 0.74 and a four-week test-retest stability of 0.64. Similarly, a one-year test-retest coefficient of 0.53 was attained for high school students, providing evidence for stability among late adolescents. Moreover, the SLSS has demonstrated good construct validity. Convergent validity for the SLSS is supported by theoretically sound correlations with other measures of self-reported and parent-reported life satisfaction, as well as with self-esteem, locus of control, and extraversion (Dew and Huebner, 1994; Gilman and Huebner, 1997; Huebner, 1991a). Evidence for discriminant validity is provided by weak or nonsignificant relationships between the SLSS and measures not theoretically related, such as intelligence, academic performance, and social desirability (Huebner and Alderman, 1993; Huebner, 1991a).

Family Support Scale (FSS) (Wills and Cleary, 1996b). This measure, developed with adolescents in grades 8–10, contains eleven items that index perceived availability of two facets of parental social support, emotional and instrumental. Emotional support is the extent to which parents offer a caring, noncritical self to the child with whom the child can share feelings, problems, and worries. Instrumental support refers to parents' provision of more concrete aid, such as transportation, information, and solutions for practical concerns. The FSS was selected as a indicator of parental warmth/involvement in order to further delineate specific subtypes of support associated with LS. Students answer each statement using a 5-point response format, on which responses vary from 1 = "not at all true to 5 = "very true".

In the current study, a correlation of 0.78 was obtained between the Emotional and Instrumental subscales, and further analyses did not support the presence of two separable factors. To avoid complications related to multicollinearity in data analyses, a score representing participants' average social support (range: 1–5) was calculated by summing responses to all items from the Emotional and Instrumental Support subscales and dividing by 11. This total parent social support variable, in which high scores are indicative of high parental support, was employed in all subsequent analyses.

The FSS has adequate internal consistency; research using this scale has reported the Cronbach alpha for the Emotional

Support subscale to be at 0.81, and $\alpha = 0.74$ for the Instrumental Support subscale (Wills, Blechman and McNamara, 1996a). Criterion validity for the FSS is provided by correlations in expected directions between this measure and adolescent substance abuse, academic competence, peer competence, adult competence, and adaptive coping (Wills et al., 1996a). This line of research also revealed that the relationship between adolescents' negative life events and substance abuse was moderated by scores on the FSS, lending validity to this scale as a measure of supportive family relationships.

Psychological Autonomy Granting (PAG) subscale of the Authoritative Parenting Measure (Steinberg, Elmen and Mounts, 1989). The nine items on the psychological autonomy scale "assess the extent to which parents employ noncoercive, democratic discipline and encourage the adolescent to express individuality within the family" (Steinberg et al., 1992: p. 1270). Students respond to each statement using a 4-point response format that ranges from 1 = "strongly disagree" to 4 = "strongly agree". All but one item is reverse scored, then items are summed so that higher scores correspond to increased parental psychological autonomy granting.

Validity for this scale is suggested by strong relationships between the Psychological Autonomy Granting scale and theoretically expected adolescent outcome variables, such as school performance and school engagement (Steinberg et al., 1992). In addition, correlations with other measures of desirable parenting characteristics (i.e., involvement in school, encouragement to succeed) lend support for criterion validity. The authors of the PAG report its internal consistency to be 0.82.

Strictness/Supervision subscale of the Authoritative Parenting Measure (Steinberg et al., 1989). The eight questions on this subscale gauge parental supervision and monitoring of adolescents' activities, as well as strictness via imposed curfews. Students indicate the latest time they are allowed out on school nights and weekends, with the choices restricted to hourly time increments, "I am not allowed out", "before 8:00", "11:00 or later", and "as late as I want". Students are also asked how much their parents try to know and really know their whereabouts. Some items are reverse scored, so that higher total scores on this measure indicate high levels of parental supervision.

Validity for this measure is suggested by theoretically sound relationships between the Strictness/Supervision Scale and adolescent outcome variables like drug use, delinquency, and grade point average (Lamborn et al., 1991). It has adequate internal consistency; previous research reported $\alpha = 0.76$ (Lamborn et al., 1991).

The Youth Self Report (YSR) form of the Child Behavior Checklist (Achenbach and Edelbrock, 1991). The YSR contains 118 items that assess eight areas of problem behavior, and provides composite scores indexing internalizing behavior, externalizing behavior, and total problems. Students rate on a 3-point scale (0 = "not true", 1 = "somewhat or sometimes true", 2 = "very true of often true") how true each item is for them now or within the past six months. For the purposes of this study, only the 61 items which comprise the internalizing (withdrawn, somatic complaints, and anxious/depressed subscales) and externalizing (delinquent behavior and aggressive behavior subscales) domains were employed. Responses on all items in each domain were summed, such that high scores reflect higher reports of problem behavior.

Validity studies have supported the usefulness of the YSR in identifying children with problem behavior. For example, adolescents referred for clinical services attained significantly higher scores on all problem subscales than nonreferred adolescents (Achenbach and Edelbrock, 1991). Furthermore, the YSR yields significant correlations with both teacher and parent reports of adolescents' problem behavior; correlations between the YSR and the Teacher Report Form of the CBCL have been reported at 0.37–0.47 for Internalizing symptoms and 0.56–0.59 for Externalizing symptoms, while correlations between the YSR and Parent Rating Form of the CBCL are reportedly between 0.38–0.42 for Internalizing and 0.43–0.49 for Externalizing. The YSR has good reliability; the one-week test-retest coefficient is 0.79.

Although not of primary interest in the current study, analyses indicated significant demographic (gender, age, race, SES) differences on this outcome measure. For example, boys reported more externalizing behaviors ($F(2, 1166) = 12.63$, $p < 0.01$), but less internalizing behaviors ($F(1, 1165) = 17.32, p < 0.01$), than girls. In the entire sample, reports of externalizing behavior showed a curvilinear pattern, peaking in middle adolescence ($F(2, 1166) = 12.63$, $p < 0.01$), while internalizing behavior was comparable across age groups, $F(2, 1165) = 2.07$, $p > 0.05$). The low SES sample reported more internalizing behavior than the average/high average SES group, $F(1, 1165) = 7.59$, $p < 0.01$. Regarding racial differences, African American students had lower externalizing scores than Caucasian and mixed-race adolescents ($F(5, 1166) = 6.99, p < 0.01$), and lower internalizing scores than Caucasian and Native American adolescents ($F(5, 1165) = 6.96, p < 0.01$).

Differences in problem behavior relevant to family structure were also noted. Adolescents living in either single-parent households headed by their fathers, or two-parent homes with their biological mother and a stepfather, had higher externalizing scores than adolescents living with both their biological parents, their mother only, or extended family members, ($F(5, 1166) = 5.00, p < 0.01$). In contrast, adolescents living with extended family members reported higher internalizing behavior than adolescents living with both biological parents, ($F(5, 1165) = 2.49, p < 0.05$).

RESULTS

Descriptive Analysis

Means and standard deviations for the entire adolescent sample, as well as for the early, middle, and late adolescent subsamples, on global adolescent LS, parental social support, psychological autonomy granting, strictness-supervision, adolescent externalizing behavior, and internalizing behavior, are presented in Table I. To further assess univariate normality, skewness and kurtosis of each of the six measures were calculated. All obtained values were within acceptable limits (between –1.0 and +1.0).

Correlational Analysis

Pearson correlations among all continuous variables included in analyses are presented for the entire sample and for each adolescent age group in Table I. As can be seen, most variables were

TABLE I

Means, standard deviations, and intercorrelations of and between target variables for early, middle, late, and total samples of adolescents

Variable	*M*	*SD*	1	2	3	4	5
Total ($n = 1188$)							
1. Strictness-supervision	20.58	4.33					
2. Social support	3.91	0.96	0.28**				
3. Autonomy granting	22.51	5.46	0.02	0.16**			
4. Life satisfaction	4.21	1.14	0.21**	0.49**	0.17**		
5. Externalizing behavior	12.97	8.15	–0.27**	–0.32**	–0.16**	–0.38**	
6. Internalizing behavior	14.10	9.62	–0.06	–0.24**	–0.23**	–0.49**	0.50**
Early ($n = 314$)							
1. Strictness-supervision	22.16	4.24					
2. Social support	4.16	0.89	0.25**				
3. Autonomy granting	21.72	5.75	0.04	0.21**			
4. Life satisfaction	4.36	1.17	0.23**	0.57**	0.20**		
5. Externalizing behavior	11.47	7.96	–0.25**	–0.31**	–0.24**	–0.42**	
6. Internalizing behavior	14.64	9.96	–0.06	–0.31**	–0.29**	–0.53**	0.60**
Middle ($n = 510$)							
1. Strictness-supervision	20.51	4.21					
2. Social support	3.88	0.93	0.28**				
3. Autonomy granting	22.55	5.19	0.05	0.14**			
4. Life satisfaction	4.15	1.14	0.18**	0.49**	0.13**		
5. Externalizing behavior	14.13	8.23	–0.31**	–0.31**	–0.12**	–0.34**	
6. Internalizing behavior	14.41	9.70	–0.09	–0.25**	–0.19**	–0.49**	0.46**
Late ($n = 364$)							
1. Strictness-supervision	19.30	4.13					
2. Social support	3.73	1.00	0.26**				
3. Autonomy granting	23.13	5.48	0.05	0.17**			
4. Life satisfaction	4.16	1.10	0.22**	0.43**	0.23**		
5. Externalizing behavior	12.63	7.97	–0.24**	–0.33**	–0.17**	–0.40**	
6. Internalizing behavior	13.17	9.16	–0.05	–0.23**	–0.23**	–0.49**	0.50**

[a]Total includes entire sample of adolescents.
[b]Early adolescents were ages 11 and 12.
[c]Middle adolescents were ages 13 to 15.
[d]Late adolescents were ages 16 to 19.
*$p < 0.05$; **$p < 0.01$.

significantly related to each other. As hypothesized, each of the authoritative parenting dimensions was positively related to adolescents' LS. The correlation (r = 0.49) between LS and parental social support suggests that adolescents' perceived emotional and instrumental support from parents is particularly related to their LS. LS was negatively related to both internalizing and externalizing behavior. Negative relationships were also revealed between all authoritative parenting dimensions and adolescent externalizing behavior, as well as between both parental social support and autonomy granting and adolescent internalizing behavior. These findings are noteworthy as clear relationships among these variables must be established as a prerequisite to analyzing the fit of subsequent mediating models. Last, as expected, there was a sizeable relationship (r = 0.50) between the two types of adolescent problem behavior.

Multiple Regression

While significant bivariate correlations established the presence of relationships between each parenting dimension and adolescent LS, a simultaneous multiple regression analysis was conducted in order to determine the total amount of variance explained in LS scores by all three authoritative parenting dimensions, as well as to evaluate the relative strength (e.g., unique variance contribution) of each parenting dimension in predicting LS when all parenting variables were considered concurrently. LS scores were regressed on the linear combination of social support, psychological autonomy granting, and strictness-supervision. The equation containing authoritative parenting dimensions accounted for 26% of the variance in LS, $F(3, 1182) = 137.10, p < 0.001$.

Beta weights (standardized multiple regression coefficients) and squared semipartial correlation coefficients (the percentage of variance in LS accounted for by a given predictor, beyond the variance accounted for by the other predictors) were then reviewed to assess the relative importance of the three parenting variables in the prediction of adolescent LS. Note that in light of significant relationships found between several demographic variables (adolescent age group, race, SES, and family structure) and LS, these variables were dummy-coded and entered first to statistically control for potential

TABLE II

Simultaneous multiple regression analysis predicting adolescent life satisfaction

Predictor	Standard $\beta^{a,b}$	sr^{2c}
Control variables		
1. Race		0.007
2. SES		0.002
3. Age		0.002
4. Family structure		0.008
Authoritative parenting dimensions		
1. Strictness-supervision	0.09*	0.006
2. Social support	0.45**	0.170
3. Psychological Autonomy granting	0.10**	0.010
		$R^2 = 0.29^d$
		Adjusted $R^2 = 0.28$

$N = 1188$.
[a]Beta weights are standardized multiple regression coefficients obtained when life satisfaction was regressed on all predictors; values cannot be obtained for categorical, dummy-coded variables.
[b]For t-tests that tested the significance of the beta weights df = 1175.
[c]Squared semipartial correlation coefficients indicate the percentage of unique variance in life satisfaction scores accounted for by a given predictor variable beyond the variance accounted for by the other six predictors.
[d]Unique variability = 0.20; shared variability = 0.085.
$^*p < 0.05$; $^{**}p < 0.001$.

confounds of these demographic factors on the relationship between authoritative parenting and LS. Beta weights and uniqueness indices are presented in Table II.

Even when an adolescent's age, SES, race, and family structure are considered, each of the three authoritative parenting dimensions is significantly related to LS (as indicated by significant beta weights). Social support demonstrated the largest beta weight at 0.45 ($p < 0.001$), while the beta weights for psychological autonomy granting and supervision were 0.10 ($p < 0.001$) and 0.09 ($p < 0.01$), respectively.

Findings regarding squared semipartial correlations matched those for beta weights, in that social support emerged as the strongest predictor of LS, accounting for approximately 17% of the variance in LS scores, beyond that explained by the remaining parenting dimensions and demographic variables. In contrast, psychological autonomy granting and strictness-supervision each accounted for only 1% of the unique variance in adolescent LS.

Adolescent Age as a Moderator in the Relationship Between Authoritative Parenting Dimensions and Adolescent Life Satisfaction

A priori, developmental differences were expected to occur in relationships involving parenting behaviors. Therefore, following guidelines suggested by Holmbeck (1997) and Cohen et al. (2003), multiple regression analyses that included interaction terms were conducted to evaluate age as a moderator in the relationship between parenting and LS. Note that age was entered in its continuous form (i.e., years old) in tests for interaction effects. LS scores were regressed on centered terms (as recommended by Cohen et al., 2003) representing adolescent age, each authoritative parenting dimension, and each interaction between adolescent age and parenting dimensions (Supervision × Age, Social Support × Age, and Autonomy Granting × Age). When predicting LS, one significant interaction was found: Parental Social Support × Age [$b = -0.07$, $t = -4.21$, $p < 0.001$, $\Delta R^2 = 0.01$], providing evidence for the moderating role of age in the relationship between parenting and LS; specifically, the influence of parental social support on adolescents' LS differs dependent on the child's age. On the other hand, no significant interactions between age and the remaining authoritative parenting dimensions were found. Thus, the influence of strictness-supervision on adolescent LS is relatively constant among adolescents of varying ages ($t = 0.47$, $p > 0.05$), as is the relationship between psychological autonomy granting and LS, $t = 1.56$, $p > 0.05$.

To interpret the interaction effect found between LS and parental social support, we followed procedures set forth in Cohen et al. (2003) and constructed simple regression lines by regressing LS on parental social support at meaningful levels of the moderator

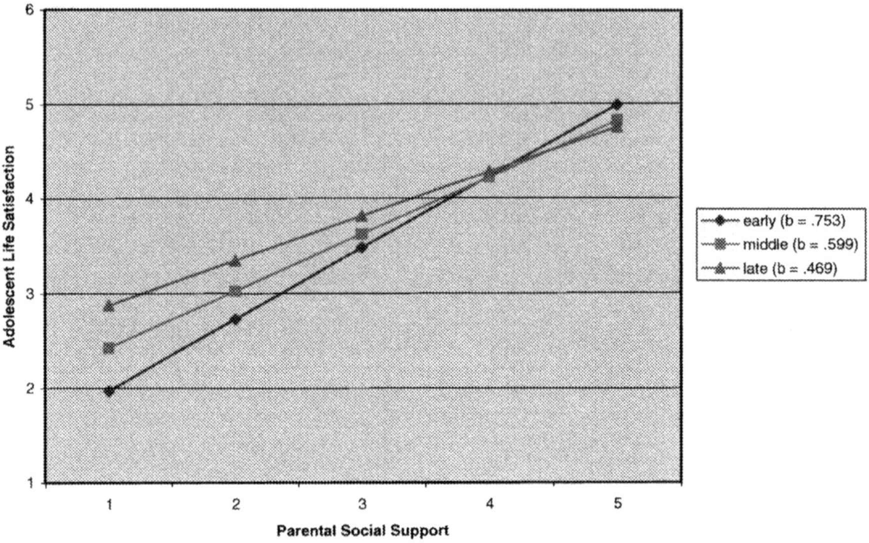

Figure 1. Interaction of parental social support with adolescent age in predicting levels of adolescent life satisfaction. Early, middle, and late refer to levels of age (i.e., adolescent age group). The slope of each line is denoted by the corresponding unstandardized regression coefficient (*b*).

(age), specifically early, middle, and late adolescence. The interaction effect is plotted in Figure 1, in which the range of social support scores is on the *x*-axis, and life satisfaction scores are on the Y-axis.

As shown in the figure, the slope of the association of social support with life satisfaction was the steepest for early adolescents ($b = 0.753$), smallest for late adolescents ($b = 0.469$, and in-between for middle adolescents ($b = 0.599$). In other words, the influence of parental social support on adolescent life satisfaction decreases as adolescents age. This finding was also indicated in additional follow-up regression analyses examining the influence of all three authoritative parenting dimensions on LS in early, middle, and late adolescents; specifically, authoritative parenting explained a greater proportion of LS in early adolescents ($R^2 = 34\%$) than in middle ($R^2 = 25\%$) or late ($R^2 = 22\%$) adolescents.

Evaluating Fit of the Mediator Model

Finally, a path model attempting to explain the significant relationships between authoritative parenting dimensions and adolescent externalizing and internalizing behavior completely through a

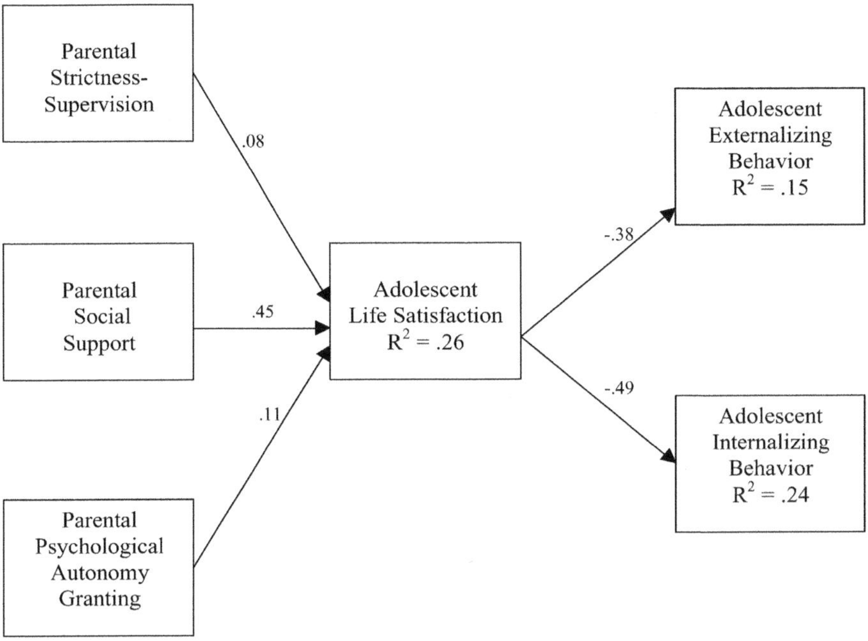

Figure 2. Hypothesized model of the relationship between authoritative parenting dimensions, adolescent life satisfaction and adolescent problem behavior in the total sample of adolescents.

mediator (life satisfaction) was tested. Data were analyzed using the SAS system's CALIS procedure. Parameter estimates were achieved via full information maximum likelihood methods. In addition, error terms between internalizing and externalizing behavior were permitted to correlate due to expected measurement effects (e.g., variables were subscales of the same measure). Figure 2 presents a graphical representation of this model, as well as obtained standardized coefficients and R^2 values.

To assess the relative fit of the sample data to this path model, the residuals and selected fit indices – Root Mean Square Residual (RMR) and Bentler's Comparative Fit Index (CFI) – were examined. Although each of the six hypothesized paths was statistically significant, suggesting important relationships between each predictor and the mediating variable, as well as between the mediator and each type of problem behavior, overall fit indices were substandard. Specifically, CFI was at 0.90, below the desired level of 0.95 or higher. The RMR value of 0.065 approached an acceptable level

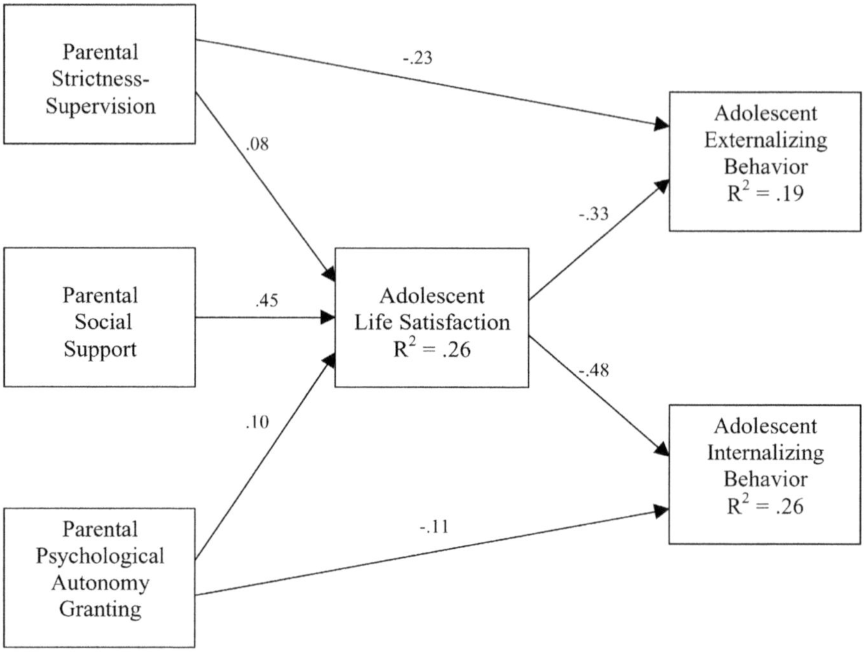

Figure 3. Revised model of the relationship between authoritative parenting dimensions, adolescent life satisfaction and adolescent problem behavior in the total sample of adolescents.

(values below 0.06 are desirable). These results suggest that LS cannot fully account for the relationships between authoritative parenting and adolescent behaviors.

To determine ways to improve model fit, residuals of the prior model were examined. Two pairs of variables possessed residual values at or above 0.15: externalizing behavior and strictness-supervision (–0.19), and internalizing behavior and psychological autonomy granting (–0.15), suggesting direct effects that were not accounted for in the original model. Therefore, a revised model that included all original paths, plus the inclusion of the direct paths just described, was tested. Results are depicted in Figure 3. Again, all paths were statistically significant. However, the revised model provided an adequate fit of the model to the data (RMR = 0.03; CFI = 0.98). In addition, all residual variances were below 0.10, suggesting that all important and necessary paths were included.

To summarize, a model that contained indirect paths from all parenting variables to problem behavior scales, as well as direct paths from parental strictness-supervision to externalizing behavior and from parental psychological autonomy granting to internalizing behavior best explains the data. LS appears to fully mediate the relationship between parental social support and problem behavior, as well as partially mediate the influence of strictness-supervision and psychological autonomy granting on problem behavior.

DISCUSSION

Consistent with previous research that suggested a general link between family and children's LS (Dew and Huebner, 1994), and a specific association between authoritative parenting and adolescents' well-being (McFarlane et al., 1995; Petito and Cummins, 2000), this study found a strong relationship between dimensions of authoritative parenting and adolescents' LS. The current study, however, clarified this general association by elucidating which particular dimensions mostly strongly relate to LS in adolescents. Results revealed that all three crucial dimensions of authoritative parenting (strictness-supervision, social support/acceptance-involvement, and psychological autonomy granting) are significantly related to LS in early, middle, and late adolescents. In other words, the more adolescents perceive their parents are monitoring their activities, providing them with emotional and instrumental support, and encouraging them to express individuality and think independently, the higher their LS is likely to be. This finding is unique to adolescence, as research with young adults demonstrated that only parental acceptance (not autonomy promotion or limit setting) provided unique contributions to college students' LS (Seibel and Johnson, 2001).

However, the current study revealed that not all authoritative parenting dimensions were of equal importance in predicting LS; when all parenting behaviors were considered simultaneously, social support emerged as the strongest pathway through which parenting influences LS. Therefore, while all authoritative parenting dimensions relate to LS, the perception of a supportive parent appeared to be most important factor in determining adolescents' LS. This finding is consistent with earlier research that found significant relationships between reciprocal social support and LS in pregnant teenagers (Stevenson et al., 1999), as well as between parents' intrinsic (i.e., emotional) support and adolescent boys' and girls' LS (Young et al., 1995).

In addition to delineating which components of parenting are crucial correlates of children's LS, this study established the important role of development in the relationship between parenting and LS. Because children from early, middle, and late adolescents were recruited for this study, important comparisons between developmental levels were made, yielding two major findings. First, the collective influence of perceived parenting behaviors on adolescents' global LS decreased across age groups. Apparently, as children age, other environmental factors partially replace the role of parents in adolescents' evaluations of their LS. For example, given that a primary goal of adolescence involves individuation and separation from family, perhaps non-familial factors such as one's self-worth and peer relations play a larger part in determining older adolescents' LS, replacing some of the prior influence of parents. The second developmental finding pertains to the influence of the particular dimensions of authoritative parenting across development. Specifically, the influence of social support on LS decreased from early to late adolescence. In other words, whether or not a parent provided resources and a comforting relationship made less of a difference to older adolescents than to younger adolescents. In contrast, associations between LS and both parental strictness-supervision and psychological autonomy granting remained relatively constant across adolescence. Although supervision decreased across developmental levels and autonomy granting increased, the extent to which these parenting behaviors related to LS was invariant. These findings emphasize the importance of considering adolescent developmental level when designing models and interventions pertaining to adolescent subjective well-being. Different factors may be more or less important depending on the youth's particular developmental level.

Just as notable is this study's finding that LS serves a functional role, mediating the relationship between authoritative parenting dimensions (particularly social support) and adolescent behavior. Support for the role of LS as a cognitive mediator is critical because it demonstrates that LS may be conceptualized as more than a epiphenomenon (Lazarus, 1991; Veenhoven, 1989). For instance, Frisch's (2000) review of LS research with adults yielded an extensive list of advantageous outcomes that stem *from* elevated LS, including increased longevity, problem-solving skills, work capacity, social and marital outcomes, and physical health. Thus, LS is more than simply a desirable attribute in and of itself, but also a prerequisite for positive psychological health. Consistent with cognitive-behavioral psychological theory, LS appears to serve as a crucial cognitive mechanism though which environmental experiences influence adolescents' behavior.

The finding that LS did not completely mediate the influence of parental strictness-supervision and psychological autonomy granting on adolescents' problem behavior is not surprising in light of findings from previous research on outcomes of parenting. Barber et al. (1994) found parental psychological control (the opposite of psychological autonomy granting) was highly correlated with children's internalizing problems, while parental behavioral control (i.e., strictness-supervision) had a strong relationship with externalizing problems. This pattern was confirmed in the current study, as direct links between supervision-externalizing behavior and autonomy granting-internalizing behavior were indicated. Nevertheless, the relative magnitude of these associations decreased each time adolescent LS was included as a mediator variable. Therefore, the current study revealed that LS partially intervenes in the strong relationships between these parent and child behaviors; LS provides a partial pathway by which supervision and autonomy granting relate to problematic behavior. Thus, other potential subjective well-being mechanisms may need to be investigated to fully account for these pathways.

Clinical implications of these results pertain to potential prevention and intervention programs aimed at developing parenting skills that promote adolescent well-being. First, the results of this study have pinpointed particular parenting behaviors that relate to adolescents' LS. Thus, designers of health promotion programs should incorporate components/elements relating to the provision of effective parental social support, in particular. Especially concerning parents with either a preference for authoritarian parenting (i.e., high supervision, low support) or limited resources and/or time to devote to parenting, it may be necessary to help these adults shift more effort from strict supervision of their youth's activities or active encouragement of their youth's individuality to a larger emphasis on the provision of emotional and instrumental support in order to maximize LS. Parents and professionals should also be aware of the increased sensitivity of younger adolescents to social support. Concerning implications for intervention and prevention of adolescent psychopathology, the mediational role of LS cannot be overemphasized. Although LS is still a desirable outcome in and of itself, this research underscores its influence on other outcomes, namely internalizing and externalizing behavior. LS may serve as a crucial psychological mechanism, linking parent behavior and youth behavior. Thus, professionals who work with adolescent clients must not only assess the "inputs" of key agents (e.g., parents) in the adolescent's life, they must also assess the nature and level of the adolescent's subjective well-being. That is, they must seek to understand how the client formulates generalized cognitive and affective interpretations of the life experiences, which predispose her/him to subsequent behavioral "outputs", such as healthy versus psychopathological behavior. Given that this research supports a mediational role of global LS judgments in the development of problem behavior, it is likely that comprehensive intervention and prevention programs may benefit from not only incorporating components aimed at enhancing environmental factors (e.g., parenting interventions), but also incorporating components aimed at enhancing adolescents' subjective well-being (e.g., life satisfaction).

Primary limitations of the current study include demographic characteristics of the sample, the social support measure employed, the cross-sectional, correlational design, and sole reliance on self-report data. Concerning the participants, the database consisted of a largely low income, African American sample from a rural environment. Although this sample afforded an abundance of data that can be used to evaluate the well-being level of an understudied population (African Americans) and racial differences in children's LS, these demographics do not adequately represent the ethnic and SES makeup of the United States, perhaps restricting the generalizability of the findings. Certain design aspects of this research also limit the confidence with which results can be interpreted.

First, the cross-sectional, correlational nature of this study prohibits causal statements regarding directionality between variables. For example, although the hypothesis that parenting behavior determines children's LS is conceivable, the notion that children with positive LS elicit desirable parenting is also plausible. Second, only adolescent self-reports of their perceptions of their parents' behaviors were used to measure authoritative parenting dimensions in this study, raising the issue of method bias. A third methodological limitation of this study pertains to the social support scale employed, which did not behave as expected since separate facets of social support were not identified.

Several directions for future research are suggested. First, research should replicate these findings with other samples. Second, in order to establish causal relations, future research should utilize longitudinal designs to assess the associations among parenting, LS and problem behaviors. Ideally, multiple informants should also be employed in order to ensure the best measurement of parenting behaviors, as actual parent behaviors may differ from adolescents' perceptions of their parents' behaviors. Third, future studies should employ scales with increased sensitivity to the types of social support offered by parents.

Despite limitations, these results are noteworthy for several reasons. First, the relationship between adolescent LS and dimensions of authoritative parenting has been clarified further. Second, the significant role of adolescent developmental level in models of LS has been highlighted. Finally, and most importantly, the functional role of LS in the linkage of parenting behavior to adolescent problem behavior has been elucidated.

ACKNOWLEDGMENTS

This article is based on Shannon M. Suldo's masters thesis at the University of South Carolina. We gratefully acknowledge the administration and students at several schools in Sumter School District 2 (Crestwood High, Ebenezer Middle, Furman Middle, Hillcrest Middle, and Lakewood High) for providing the database utilized in this study. Also, we thank Jennifer Clayton, Julie

Seligson, Laura Smith, Robyn Waizenhofer, and Jeff White for their help with data collection.

REFERENCES

Achenbach, T.M. and C.S. Edelbrock: 1991, Child Behavior Checklist and Youth Self-Report (Author, Burlington, VT).

Adelman, H., L. Taylor and P. Nelson: 1989, 'Minors' dissatisfaction with their life circumstances', Child Psychiatry and Human Development 20(2), pp. 135–147.

Barber, B.K., J.E. Olsen and S.C. Shagle: 1994, 'Associations between parental psychological and behavioral control and youth internalized and externalized behavior', Child Development 65, pp. 1120–1136.

Baron, R.M. and D.A. Kenny: 1986, 'The moderator-mediator variable distinction in social psychology research: Conceptual, strategic, and statistical considerations', Journal of Personality and Social Psychology 51, pp. 1173–1182.

Baumrind, D.: 1991, 'The influence of parenting style on adolescent competence and substance use', Journal of Early Adolescence 11, pp. 56–95.

Bender, T.A.: 1997, 'Assessment of subjective well-being during childhood and adolescence', in G.D. Phye (ed.), Handbook of Classroom Assessment: Learning, Achievement, and Adjustment (Academic Press, San Diego, CA), pp. 199–225.

Brendgen, M., F. Vitaro and W.M. Bukowski: 1998, 'Affiliation with delinquent friends: Contributions of parents, self-esteem, delinquent behavior, and rejection by peers', Journal of Early Adolescence 18(3), pp. 244–265.

Burke, R.J. and T. Weir: 1978, 'Benefits to adolescents of informal helping relationships with their parents and peers', Psychological Reports 42(3), pp. 1175–1184.

Burke, R.J. and T. Weir: 1979, 'Helping responses of parents and peers and adolescent well-being', The Journal of Psychology 102(1), pp. 49–62.

Cobb, N.J.: 1998, Adolescence: Continuity, Change, and Diversity, 3rd edition (Mayfield Publishing Company, Mountain View, CA).

Cohen, J., P. Cohen, S.G. West and L.S. Aiken: 2003, Applied Multiple Regression/Correlation Analysis for the Behavioral Sciences, 3rd edition (Erlbaum, Mahwah, NJ).

Demo, D.H. and A.C. Acock: 1996, 'Family structure, family process, and adolescent well-being', Journal of Research on Adolescence 6(4), pp. 457–488.

Dew, T. and E.S. Huebner: 1994, 'Adolescents' perceived quality of life: An exploratory investigation', Journal of School Psychology 33(2), pp. 185–199.

Diener, E.: 1994, 'Assessing subjective well-being: Progress and opportunities', Social Indicators Research 31, pp. 103–157.

Diener, E.: 2000, 'Subjective well-being: The science of happiness and a proposal for a national index', American Psychologist 55(1), pp. 34–43.

DuBois, D.L., R.D. Felner, M.D. Sherman and C.A. Bull: 1994, 'Socioenvironmental experiences, self-esteem, and emotional/behavioral problems in early adolescence', American Journal of Community Psychology 22(3), pp. 371–397.

Frisch, M.B.: 2000, 'Improving mental and physical health care through quality of life therapy and assessment', in E. Diener and D.R. Rahtz (eds.), Advances in Quality of Life Theory and Research (Kluwer Academic Press: Great Britain), pp. 207–241.

Gilman, R. and E.S. Huebner: 1997, 'Children's reports of their life satisfaction', School Psychology International 18, pp. 229–243.

Gray, M.R. and L. Steinberg: 1999, 'Unpacking authoritative parenting: Reassessing a multidimensional construct', Journal of Marriage and the Family 61, pp. 574–587.

Grossman, M. and K.M. Rowat: 1995, 'Parental relationships, coping strategies, received support and well-being in adolescents of separated or divorced and married parents', Research in Nursing & Health 18, pp. 249–261.

Heaven, P.C.L.: 1989, 'Extraversion, neuroticism, and satisfaction with life among adolescents', Personality and Individual Differences 10(5), pp. 489–492.

Holmbeck, G.N.: 1997, 'Toward terminological, conceptual, and statistical clarity in the study of mediators and moderators: Examples from the child-clinical and pediatric psychology literatures', Journal of Clinical and Consulting Psychology 65, pp. 599–610.

Homel, R. and A. Burns: 1989, 'Environmental quality and the wellbeing of children', Social Indicators Research 21, pp. 133–158.

Huebner, E.S.: 1991a, 'Correlates of life satisfaction in children', School Psychology Quarterly 6(2), pp. 103–111.

Huebner, E.S.: 1991b, 'Initial development of the Students' Life Satisfaction Scale', School Psychology International 12, pp. 231–240.

Huebner, E.S. and G.L. Alderman: 1993, 'Convergent and discriminant validation of a children's life satisfaction scale: Its relationship to self- and teacher-reported psychological problems and school functioning', Social Indicators Research 30, pp. 71–82.

Lamborn, S.D., N.S. Mounts, L. Steinberg and S.M. Dornbusch: 1991, 'Patterns of competence and adjustment among adolescents from authoritative, authoritarian, indulgent, and neglectful families', Child Development 62, pp. 1049–1065.

Lazurus, R.S.: 1991, Emotion and Adaptation (Oxford University Press, New York).

Leung, J. P. and K. Leung: 1992, 'Life satisfaction, self-concept, and relationship with parents in adolescence', Journal of Youth and Adolescence 21(6), pp. 653–665.

Leung, J.P. and L.W. Zhang: 2000, 'Modeling life satisfaction of Chinese adolescents in Hong Kong', International Journal of Behavioral Development 24, pp. 99–104.

Liebkind, K. and I. Jasinskaja-Lahti: 2000, 'Acculturation and psychological well-being among immigrant adolescents in Finland: A comparative study of adolescents from different cultural backgrounds', Journal of Adolescent Research 15(4), pp. 446–469.

Man, P.: 1991, 'The influence of peers and parents on youth life satisfaction in Hong Kong', Social Indicators Research 24, pp. 347–365.

McCullough, G., E.S. Huebner and J.E. Laughlin: 2000, 'Life events, self-concept, and adolescents positive subjective well-being', Psychology in the Schools 37, pp. 1–10.

McFarlane, A.H., A. Bellissimo and G.R. Norman: 1995, 'Family structure, family functioning and adolescent well-being: The transcendent influence of parental style', Journal of Child Psychology and Psychiatry 36(5), pp. 847–864.

Patterson, G.R. and M. Stouthamer-Loeber: 1984, 'The correlation of family management practices and delinquency', Child Development 55(4), pp. 1299–1307.

Petito, F. and R.A. Cummins: 2000, 'Quality of life in adolescence: The role of perceived control, parenting style and social support', Behaviour Change 17, pp. 196–207.

Sam, D.L.: 1998, 'Predicting life satisfaction among adolescents from immigrant families in Norway', Ethnicity & Health 3, pp. 5–18.

Sastre, M.T.M. and G. Ferriere: 2000, 'Family "decline" and the subjective well-being of adolescent', Social Indicators Research 49, pp. 69–82.

Schaefer, E.S.: 1965, 'Children's reports of parental behavior: An inventory', Child Development 36, pp. 413–424.

Seibel, F.L and W.B. Johnson: 2001, 'Parental control, trait anxiety, and satisfaction with life in college students', Psychological Reports 88, pp. 473–480.

Shagle, S.C. and B.K. Barber: 1995, 'A social-ecological analysis of adolescent suicidal ideation', American Journal of Orthopsychiatry 65, pp. 114–124.

Shek, D.T.L.: 1997a, 'The relation of family functioning to adolescent psychological well-being, school adjustment, and problem behavior', The Journal of Genetic Psychology 158(4), pp. 467–479.

Shek, D.T.L.: 1997b, 'The relation of parent-adolescent conflict to adolescent psychological well-being, school adjustment, and problem behavior', Social Behavior and Personality 25(3), pp. 277–290.

Shek, D.T.L.: 1999, 'Individual and dyadic predictors of family functioning in a chinese context', The American Journal of Family Therapy 27, pp. 49–61.

Smollar, J. and J. Youniss: 1989, 'Transformations in adolescents' perceptions of parents', International Journal of Behavioral Development 12(1), pp. 71–84.

Stein, J.A. and M.D. Newcomb: 1999, 'Adult outcomes of adolescent conventional and agentic orientations: A 20-year longitudinal study', Journal of Early Adolescence 19(1), pp. 39–65.

Steinberg, L., J.D. Elman and M.S. Mounts: 1989, 'Authoritative parenting, psychosocial maturity, and academic success among adolescents', Child Development 60, pp. 1424–1436.

Steinberg, L., S.D. Lamborn, S.M. Dornbusch and N. Darling: 1992, 'Impact of parenting practices on adolescent achievement: Authoritative parenting, school involvement, and encouragement to succeed', Child Development 63, pp. 1266–1281.

Steinberg, L., N.S. Mounts, S.D. Lamborn and S.M. Dornbusch: 1991, 'Authoritative parenting and adolescent adjustment across varied ecological niches', Journal of Research on Adolescence 1(1), pp. 19–36.

Stevenson, W., K.I. Maton and D.M. Teti: 1999, 'Social support, relationship quality, and well-being among pregnant adolescents', Journal of Adolescence 22, pp. 109–121.

Veenhoven, R.: 1989, How Harmful Is Happiness? (Universitaire Pers Rotterdam, Rotterdam).

Wills, T.A., E.A. Blechman and G. McNamara: 1996a, 'Family support, coping, and competence', in E.M. Hetherington and E.A. Blechman (eds.), Stress, Coping, and Resiliency in Children and Families (Lawrence Erlbaum Associates, Mahwah, NJ), pp. 107–133.

Wills, T.A. and S.D. Cleary: 1996b, 'How are social support effects mediated: A test for parental support and adolescent substance use', Journal of Personality and Social Psychology 71, pp. 937–952.

Wilson, S.M., C.S. Henry and G.W. Peterson: 1997, 'Life satisfaction among low-income rural youth from Appalachia', Journal of Adolescence 20, pp. 443–459.

Wong, M.M. and M. Csikszentmihalyi: 1991, 'Motivation and academic achievement: The effects of personality traits and the quality of experience', Journal of Personality 59(3), pp. 539–574.

Young, M.H., B.C. Miller, M.C. Norton and E.J. Hill: 1995, 'The effect of parental supportive behaviors on life satisfaction of adolescent offspring', Journal of Marriage and Family 57, pp. 813–822.

Zimmerman, M.A., D.A. Salem and K.I. Maton: 1995, 'Family structure and psychosocial correlates among urban African-American adolescent males', Child Development 66, pp. 1598–1613.

Department of Psychology
University of South Carolina
Columbia, SC 29208
USA
E-mail: huebner@sc.edu or *suldo@sc.edu*

Social Indicators Research Series

1. V. Møller (ed.): *Quality of Life in South Africa.* 1997 ISBN 0-7923-4797-8
2. G. Baechler: *Violence Through Environmental Discrimination.* Causes, Rwanda Arena, and Conflict Model. 1999 ISBN 0-7923-5495-8
3. P. Bowles and L.T. Woods (eds.): *Japan after the Economic Miracle.* In Search of New Directories. 1999 ISBN 0-7923-6031-1
4. E. Diener and D.R. Rahtz (eds.): *Advances in Quality of Life Theory and Research.* Volume I. 1999 ISBN 0-7923-6060-5
5. Kwong-leung Tang (ed.): *Social Development in Asia.* 2000 ISBN 0-7923-6256-X
6. M.M. Beyerlein (ed.): *Work Teams: Past, Present and Future.* 2000 ISBN 0-7923-6699-9
7. A. Ben-Arieh, N.H. Kaufman, A.B. Andrews, R. Goerge, B.J. Lee, J.L. Aber (eds.): *Measuring and Monitoring Children's Well-Being.* 2001 ISBN 0-7923-6789-8
8. M.J. Sirgy: *Handbook of Quality-of-Life Research. An Ethical Marketing Perspective.* 2001 ISBN 1-4020-0172-X
9. G. Preyer and M. Bös (eds.): *Borderlines in a Globalized World.* New Perspectives in a Sociology of the World-System. 2002 ISBN 1-4020-0515-6
10. V. Nikolic-Ristanovic: *Social Change, Gender and Violence: Post-communist and war affected societies.* 2002 ISBN 1-4020-0726-4
11. M.R. Hagerty, J. Vogel and V. Møller: *Assessing Quality of Life and Living Conditions to Guide National Policy.* 2002 ISBN 1-4020-0727-2
12. M.J. Sirgy: *The Psychology of Quality of Life.* 2002 ISBN 1-4020-0800-7
13. S. McBride, L. Dobuzinskis, M. Griffin Cohen and J. Busumtwi-Sam (eds.): *Global Instability.* Uncertainty and new visions in political economy. 2002 ISBN 1-4020-0946-1
14. Doh. Chull Shin, C.P. Rutkowski and Chong-Min Park (eds.): *The Quality of Life in Korea.* Comparative and Dynamic Perspectives. 2003 ISBN 1-4020-0947-X
15. W. Glatzer: *Rich and Poor.* Disparities, Perceptions, Concomitants. 2002 ISBN 1-4020-1012-5
16. E. Gullone and R.A. Cummins (eds.): *The Universality of Subjective Wellbeing Indicators.* A Multi-disciplinary and Multi-national Perspective. 2002 ISBN 1-4020-1044-3
17. B.D. Zumbo (ed.): *Advances in Quality of Life Research 2001.* 2003 ISBN 1-4020-1100-8
18. J. Vogel, T. Theorell, S. Svallfors, H.-H. Noll and B. Christoph: *European Welfare Production.* Institutional Configuration and Distributional Outcome. 2003 ISBN 1-4020-1149-0
19. A.C. Michalos: *Essays on the Quality of Life.* 2003 ISBN 1-4020-1342-6
20. M.J. Sirgy, D. Rahtz and A.C. Samli (eds.): *Advances in Quality-of-Life Theory and Research.* 2003 ISBN 1-4020-1474-0
21. M. Fine-Davis, J. Fagnani, D. Giovannini, L. Højgaard and H. Clarke: *Fathers and Mothers: Dilemmas of the Work-Life Balance.* 2004 ISBN 1-4020-1807-X
22. M.J. Sirgy, D.R. Rahtz and D.J. Lee (eds.): *Community Quality-of-Life Indicators.* Best Cases. 2004 ISBN 1-4020-2201-8

23. A. Dannerbeck, F. Casas, M. Sadurni and G. Coenders (eds.): *Quality-of-Life Research on Children and Adolescents.* 2004 ISBN 1-4020-2311-1

KLUWER ACADEMIC PUBLISHERS – DORDRECHT / LONDON / BOSTON

9 781402 023118

GPSR Compliance

The European Union's (EU) General Product Safety Regulation (GPSR) is a set of rules that requires consumer products to be safe and our obligations to ensure this.

If you have any concerns about our products, you can contact us on ProductSafety@springernature.com

In case Publisher is established outside the EU, the EU authorized representative is:

Springer Nature Customer Service Center GmbH
Europaplatz 3
69115 Heidelberg, Germany

Batch number: 10823959

Printed by Printforce, the Netherlands